Best of Fives
for Dentistry

Third Edition

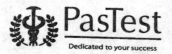

PasTest
Dedicated to your success

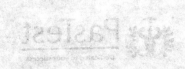

Best of Fives for Dentistry

Third Edition

Douglas Hammond
BDS (Wales) MFGDP (UK) MBBS MRCS

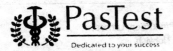

PasTest
Dedicated to your success

© 2014 PASTEST LTD
Egerton Court
Parkgate Estate
Knutsford
Cheshire
WA16 8DX

Telephone: 01565 752000

First Published 2006
Second Edition Published 2009, Reprinted 2011
Third Edition Published 2014

ISBN: 1905635 88 5
       978 1905635 88 7

A catalogue record for this book is available from the British Library.

The information contained within this book was obtained by the author from reliable sources. However, while every effort has been made to ensure its accuracy, no responsibility for loss, damage or injury occasioned to any person acting or refraining from action as a result of information contained herein can be accepted by the publishers or author.

PasTest Revision Books and Intensive Courses

PasTest has been established in the field of undergraduate and postgraduate medical education since 1972, providing revision books and intensive study courses for doctors preparing for their professional examinations.

Books, courses and online revision available for:
Medical undergraduates, MRCGP, MRCP Parts 1 and 2, MRCPCH Parts 1 and 2, MRCS, MRCOG, DRCOG, DCH, FRCA, Dentistry.

For further details contact:
PasTest, Freepost, Knutsford, Cheshire WA16 7BR

Tel: 01565 752000 Fax: 01565 650264
www.pastest.co.uk enquiries@pastest.co.uk

Text prepared in the UK by Carnegie Book Production, Lancaster
Printed and bound in the UK by Page Bros, Norwich

Contents

About the Author

Douglas Hammond BDS (Wales) MFGDP (UK) MBBS (UCL and Royal Free Medical School) MRCS (Royal College of Surgeons London)

Douglas graduated from Cardiff Dental Hospital and completed various hospital and practice jobs. He then began working as a part-time Lecturer in Oral and Maxillofacial Surgery at the Royal London Hospital in 2002, whilst embarking on a medical degree at University College London. He qualified and then completed his House officer and Senior House Officer jobs at Southampton General Hospital. He achieved his MRCS in November 2008 and has begun as a Specialist Registrar in Oral and Maxillofacial Surgery on the West Midlands rotation.

Introduction

This book has been designed to test the knowledge of final year dental students, those sitting the MJDF, and also those attempting the ORE. The questions closely resemble the type and level of knowledge required to pass these examinations. The feedback that I have received is extremely positive with regard to this. I hope that this third edition of *Best of Fives for Dentistry*, with several new questions and answers, helps to increase the knowledge base of the reader.

1
Oral Medicine

1.1 Which one of the following would be the most appropriate initial course of action in an 80-year-old man presenting with an ulcerated lesion in the anterior denture-bearing region?

A Construct new dentures

B Easing of dentures

C Excisional biopsy

D Incisional biopsy

E Urgent referral to maxillofacial unit

1.2 Which area of the mouth is most commonly affected by burning mouth syndrome?

A Hard palate

B Lips

C Retromolar region

D Soft palate

E Tongue

1.3 Which one of the following is most commonly associated with an oral diagnosis of Crohn disease?

A Clusters of ulceration

B Dysaesthesia of the tongue

C Mucosal blistering

D Mucosal tags

E Swollen lips

1.4 Which one of the following medications is most likely to be associated with a dry mouth?

A Aspirin

B Atenolol

C Bendroflumethazide

D Captopril

E Nicorandil

1.1   B

Any ulcerated lesion under a denture is most commonly denture trauma. Therefore the denture should be eased, and the patient reviewed at 2 weeks. If the lesion has not improved, an urgent referral is appropriate.

1.2   E

'Burning' is most frequently reported in the tongue region (80% of patients with burning mouth syndrome). Most patients who develop burning mouth syndrome are postmenopausal women. The female:male ratio with burning mouth syndrome is 7:1. This is a relatively common problem seen all over the world, eg in the Netherlands, patients with burning mouth syndrome have formed a support group. It seems to be a condition that affects people of all races and all socioeconomic backgrounds.

1.3   D

Although ulceration, swollen lips and rarely dysaesthesia can be present in patients who have Crohn disease, it is the tissue diagnosis from mucosal tags that will be diagnostic.

1.4   C

Bendroflumethazide is a thiazide diuretic, which is mainly used to treat hypertension. Diuretics such as bendroflumethiazide make you lose circulating volume. Occasionally the patient may lose too much and become dehydrated. The patient should let his or her doctor know if he or she feels constantly thirsty, has a dry mouth or has skin that looks and feels dry.

1.5   A patient presents with angular cheilitis, and you decide to perform
       some haematological investigations. Which one of the following
       tests is not relevant to angular cheilitis?

       A   Full blood count

       B   Fasting venous glucose

       C   Vitamin B$_{12}$

       D   Liver function tests

       E   Ferritin

1.6   Which one of the following drugs is inappropriate for the treatment
       of angular cheilitis?

       A   Aciclovir

       B   Nystatin

       C   Miconazole

       D   Fluconazole

       E   Amphotericin

1.7   Target lesions are associated with which one of the following
       conditions?

       A   Stevens–Johnson syndrome

       B   Major aphthous stomatitis

       C   Pemphigus

       D   Pemphigoid

       E   Syphilis

1.5   D

Some studies have shown that 50% of patients with angular cheilitis have haematological abnormalities. Anaemia and diabetes are the most common of these. The liver function tests are irrelevant.

1.6   A

Aciclovir is an antiviral agent, and it is used mainly for human herpes virus infections. Nystatin, amphotericin and miconazole are used topically. Amphotericin can be used systemically, but it has many side effects, so it should not be used systemically for a minor infection such as angular cheilitis. Fluconazole, however, can be used systemically.

1.7   A

Stevens–Johnson syndrome produces target lesions on the skin which look like 'bull's eyes'. This reaction is frequently caused by drug reactions, especially to sulphonamides. Patients can be systemically very unwell, and more often than not require admission.

1.8 **What is the male to female ratio of the prevalence of recurrent aphthous ulceration/stomatitis?**

    A 3:1

    B 2:1

    C 1:1

    D 1:2

    E 1:3

1.9 **What is the best treatment for mumps?**

    A Aciclovir

    B Prednisolone

    C Augmentin

    D Clarithromycin

    E Nothing

1.10 **What is the male to female ratio of patients with 'burning mouth syndrome'?**

    A 7:1

    B 3:1

    C 1:1

    D 1:3

    E 1:7

1.8 **C**

Recurrent aphthous ulceration occurs equally among males and females.

1.9 **E**

Mumps is a self-resolving condition, and requires no treatment.

1.10 **E**

Females are far more likely than males to report burning mouth syndrome.

1.11 What is the mean age of presentation in burning mouth syndrome?

  A   18 years

  B   25 years

  C   40 years

  D   60 years

  E   80 years

1.12 A child of 14 months presents with blood-crusted lips, pyrexia and widespread oral ulceration. What is the most likely diagnosis?

  A   Teething

  B   Traumatic injury

  C   Primary herpetic gingivostomatitis

  D   Hand, foot and mouth

  E   Human papilloma virus

1.13 Which one of the following does not cause the reactivation of herpes simplex infection?

  A   Stress

  B   Sunlight

  C   Immunosuppression

  D   Local trauma

  E   Dental caries

1.11 D

Burning mouth syndrome is far more prevalent in women than in men, has a mean age of presentation of 60 years, and is rarely seen in people younger than 45 years. There are many causes of burning mouth syndrome. These include vitamin B complex deficiency, haematological disorders, undiagnosed type 2 diabetes, xerostomia, parafunctional habits, poorly constructed dentures, cancerphobia, anxiety, depression, climacteric and allergy. It is important to investigate these patients haematologically and psychologically.

1.12 C

A traumatic injury would be possible, but it is unlikely as the child has pyrexia. Teething would not cause blood-crusted lips. Human papilloma virus does not cause this. The treatment for primary herpetic gingivostomatitis is aciclovir, antiseptic mouthwash, and paracetamol to reduce the pyrexia. The child should be discouraged from touching the lesion, and their fluid intake increased.

1.13 E

The common triggers for reactivation of herpes simplex are stress, local trauma, exposure to sunlight or cold, menstruation, systemic upset and immunosuppression.

1.14 A 12-year-old child who has had chickenpox previously presents with vesicles in and around his left ear, hearing loss and some facial nerve weakness. What is the diagnosis?

    A   Herpes simplex 1 reactivation

    B   Herpes simplex 2 reactivation

    C   Ramsay–Hunt syndrome

    D   Coxsackie viral infection

    E   Infectious mononucleosis

1.15 What is the usual prescription of aciclovir given to patients with acute herpes simplex infection?

    A   200 mg twice daily for 5–10 days

    B   200 mg three times daily for 5–10 days

    C   200 mg four times daily for 5–10 days

    D   200 mg five times daily for 5–10 days

    E   200 mg six times daily for 5–10 days

1.16 A 70-year-old patient presents with systemic upset, a unilateral headache around the temporal region, and a severe cramp-like pain when the patient begins to chew. They have never had any symptoms like this before. What is your diagnosis?

    A   Paroxysmal facial hemicrania

    B   Giant cell arteritis

    C   Periodic migrainous neuralgia

    D   Salivary calculi

    E   Trigeminal neuralgia

1.14 C

Ramsay–Hunt syndrome originates in the geniculate ganglion of the seventh cranial nerve and is associated with varicella zoster infection. Treatment is usually with steroids and antivirals, to reduce the chance of permanent hearing loss.

1.15 D

Aciclovir is one of the unusual medicines required to be taken five times daily.

1.16 B

This is a classic presentation of giant cell arteritis, which can be a medical emergency. It requires the prompt administration of prednisolone to prevent the onset of blindness.

1.17   What would be the best blood test to aid your diagnosis in
        Question 1.16?

A   Full blood count

B   Liver function tests

C   Erythrocyte sedimentation rate (ESR)

D   Vitamin B_{12}

E   International normalised ratio (INR)

1.18   A 15-year-old patient presents with pyrexia, sore throat and bilateral
        parotitis. However, on palpation of the parotids the saliva is clear,
        and there is no xerostomia. What is your most likely diagnosis?

A   Measles

B   Mumps

C   Bacterial parotitis

D   Sjögren's disease

E   Cytomegalovirus

1.19   Which one of the following viruses is associated with Kaposi's
        sarcoma?

A   Human herpes virus 1

B   Human herpes virus 2

C   Varicella zoster virus

D   Cytomegalovirus

E   Human herpes virus 8

1.17   C

ESR is a marker of inflammation, and is markedly raised in patients with giant cell arteritis.

1.18   B

Sjögren's disease is possible, however there is no reduced saliva flow. Bacterial parotitis would produce a pus-filled saliva, and therefore it would not be clear. It would also be unusual to have bilateral bacterial parotitis. Mumps is the most common cause of bilateral parotitis. It usually settles down after 2 weeks, but patients must be aware that the complications of mumps include orchitis or oophoritis, leading to infertility. Mumps is on the increase as parents are reluctant to vaccinate their children with the MMR (measles, mumps, rubella) vaccine because of the controversy surrounding it.

1.19   E

Kaposi's sarcoma is an acquired immune deficiency syndrome (AIDS)-related illness associated with human herpes virus 8. It has three forms: classic, endemic and epidemic.

1.20 A patient presents with a unilateral, electric shock-like pain along the course of the mandible. He says it happens when he shaves, and it is the worst pain he has ever had. What is your likely diagnosis?

A Temporomandibular joint dysfunction

B Trigeminal neuralgia

C Dental abscess

D Parotitis

E Paroxysmal facial hemicrania

1.21 What would be the best medication for the condition in Question 1.20?

A Dothiepin

B Fluoxetine

C Carbamazepine

D Prednisolone

E Amitriptyline

1.22 Which one of the following blood tests is important when monitoring patients taking carbamazepine?

A Vitamin B_{12}

B Ferritin

C Erythrocyte sedimentation rate

D Liver function tests

E Serum folate

1.20   B

This is the classic description of trigeminal neuralgia.

1.21   C

Carbamazepine is the treatment of choice for trigeminal neuralgia. Patients are usually started on 100 mg three times daily and then require an increase in the dose after a month or two to 200 mg three times daily to a maximum of 800 mg three times daily. These patients require regular monitoring. Prednisolone is a steroid, used for many conditions but not for neuralgia. The other drugs are more effective in patients with atypical facial pain.

1.22   D

Carbamazepine is metabolised in the liver and can lead to altered liver function and can cause drug-induced inflammation of the liver (hepatitis). It can also cause aplastic anaemia in a few patients, so a full blood count is also useful.

1.23   An 18-year-old girl presents with a grossly enlarged lower lip, angular cheilitis, full-width gingivitis, mucosal tags and cobblestone mucosae. What is the most likely diagnosis?

   A   Allergic reaction leading to anaphylaxis

   B   Lichenoid reaction

   C   Erythema multiforme

   D   Orofacial granulomatosis (OFG)

   E   Lichen planus

1.24   Which gastrointestinal condition is commonly associated with orofacial granulomatosis?

   A   Ulcerative colitis

   B   Crohn's disease

   C   Coeliac disease

   D   Irritable bowel disease

   E   Hirschsprung's disease

1.25   In patients who truly have an allergic reaction to local anaesthetic, which one of the following is the most likely cause?

   A   Lidocaine

   B   Adrenaline

   C   Octapressin

   D   Methylparaben

   E   Sodium chloride

1.23 D

An incisional biopsy down to muscle will show that this patient has non-caseating granulomas and lymphoedema, which are indicative of OFG. It is associated with reactions to cinnamon and benzoates, and patients with OFG frequently have a large intake of these substances. Patients with OFG also show a tendency to have atopic conditions such as eczema and asthma.

1.24 B

Crohn's disease has the same histological features as OFG and is present in 12% of patients with OFG.

1.25 D

Methylparaben is the preservative in local anaesthetics, and is the most common cause of an allergic reaction in patients. Occasionally sodium bisulphite is used as a preservative and this too can cause an allergic reaction. It would be highly unlikely that a patient is allergic to adrenaline as the body produces it.

1.26 Which one of the following does not predispose a patient to candidosis?

A Currently taking a broad-spectrum antibiotic

B Taking prednisolone daily

C Agranulocytosis

D Stress

E Folic acid deficiency

1.27 What condition is Wickham's striae associated with?

A Pseudomembranous candidosis

B Chronic hyperplastic candidosis

C Lichenoid reactions

D Lichen planus

E White sponge naevus

1.28 Which one of the following autoantibodies is not associated with Sjögren's syndrome?

A Anti-Ro

B Anti-La

C Rheumatoid factor

D Anti-nuclear antibodies

E Anti-Smith antibodies

1.26   D

All of the others are predisposing factors for candidosis.

1.27   D

Lichen planus is a systemic as well as an oral disease. It is actually more commonly found extra-orally. Wickham's striae are irregular, itchy, white streaks on the flexor surfaces of the forearms, elbows and ankles. We must remember that patients have bodies and not just mouths! Looking at the rest of the body can aid our diagnosis.

1.28   E

Anti-Smith antibodies are associated with systemic lupus erythematosus. It is important to know which antibodies are associated with Sjögren's syndrome. It is a viva favourite!

1.29 Sjögren's syndrome is associate with other autoimmune diseases (acronym CREST). Which one of the following is not involved in CREST syndrome?

    A   Calcinosis

    B   Raynaud's phenomenon

    C   Rheumatic fever

    D   Oesophageal dysmotility

    E   Telangiectasia

1.30 A 75-year-old lady with a history of gastric cancer who has been clear of the disease for 25 years presents to you with a red, raw beefy tongue, oral ulceration, tachycardia, numbness in the extremities and an unusual gait. What would be your most likely diagnosis?

    A   Iron-deficiency anaemia

    B   Vitamin B_{12} deficiency

    C   Recurrence of gastric cancer

    D   Brain tumour

    E   Alzheimer's disease

1.31 If you suspect vitamin B_{12} deficiency in a patient, and you want to know whether lack of intrinsic factor is the cause, which test would you perform?

    A   Full blood count

    B   Red cell folate

    C   Schilling's test

    D   Ferritin

    E   Bence Jones protein

1.29 C

Patients with Sjögren's syndrome frequently have other autoimmune disorders. Xerostomia is the most common presentation, but they may have other systemic diseases which are linked to this. It is important to ask them about having cold fingers, difficulty swallowing and arthritis, and to look for telangiectasia.

1.30 B

Having had a gastric cancer previously, it is likely that the patient has a reduced amount of intrinsic factor, and therefore reduced absorption of vitamin B_{12}. As she has been clear of cancer for 25 years it is unlikely that she has had a recurrence or has a brain tumour. Vitamin B_{12} deficiency leads to the classic red, raw beefy tongue, oral ulceration and peripheral neuropathy.

1.31 C

For Schilling's test, after an overnight fast, the patient is given an injection of non-radiolabelled vitamin B_{12} to saturate the body's stores. The patient then takes an oral vitamin B_{12} dose labelled with cobalt 58, followed by an oral dose of vitamin B_{12} and intrinsic factor labelled with cobalt 57. Urine is collected over 24 hours to measure the levels of the isotopes present in it. From the urinary levels it can be worked out if the cause is a lack of intrinsic factor. Bence Jones proteins are measured in multiple myeloma.

1.32 Which one of the following drugs does not cause a lichenoid
reaction?

A   β-Blockers

B   Gold

C   Allopurinol

D   Nifedipine

E   Anti-malarials

1.33 Which one of the following conditions/lesions is not caused by
viruses?

A   Koplik's spots

B   Herpetiform ulceration

C   Herpes labialis

D   Hand, foot and mouth disease

E   Herpangina

1.34 Which one of the following is not a type of lichen planus?

A   Plaque-like

B   Atrophic

C   Hyperplastic

D   Erosive

E   Reticular

1.32   D

Nifedipine causes gingival hyperplasia not lichenoid reaction.

1.33   B

Herpetiform ulceration means that the ulcers look like herpes but are not actually caused by herpes virus. Hand, foot and mouth disease and herpangina are caused by coxsackie virus. Koplik's spots are associated with measles.

1.34   C

All others are types of lichen planus.

1.35 In which age group does lichen planus usually occur?

A   0–18 years

B   18–30 years

C   30–50 years

D   50–70 years

E   70+ years

1.36 If temporal arteritis is left untreated, what is the most serious complication?

A   Blindness

B   Deafness

C   Anosmia

D   Paralysis of the muscles of mastication

E   Loss of taste

1.37 Which one of the following is not described in a classical history of trigeminal neuralgia?

A   10/10 pain

B   Shooting or electric shock-like pain

C   There is a trigger factor

D   It is bilateral

E   Occurs in the region of the mandibular branch of the trigeminal nerve

1.35   C

About half of people with a lichen planus skin rash develop white streaks on the inside of the cheeks, gums or tongue. This is usually painless and not itchy. It may not be noticed unless looked for. Sometimes lichen planus of the mouth occurs without any skin rash. Lichen planus can also cause ulcers in the mouth but this is uncommon. If ulcers do occur they can be very sore and unpleasant, and hot or spicy foods are especially difficult to eat. Mouth ulcers can occur with or without the skin rash. In some cases, the gums become red and sore.

1.36   A

The most serious complication of temporal arteritis is blindness.

1.37   D

Trigeminal neuralgia is a neuropathic disorder of the trigeminal nerve that causes episodes of intense pain in the eyes, lips, nose, scalp, forehead and jaw. The pain is unilateral. It is estimated that 1 in 15 000 people have from trigeminal neuralgia, although the numbers may be considerably higher due to frequent misdiagnosis. Trigeminal neuralgia usually develops after the age of 50, more commonly in women, although there have been cases of patients as young as 3 years of age. The condition can bring about stabbing, mind-numbing, electric shock-like pain from just a finger's glance of the cheek.

1.38 **To which virus family does varicella zoster belong?**

   A Coxsackie

   B Herpes

   C Hepadnavirus

   D Parvovirus

   E Respiratory syncytial virus (RSV)

1.39 **A 7-year-old boy presents with bilateral parotitis. What is the most likely diagnosis?**

   A Sjögren's syndrome

   B CREST

   C Salivary calculi

   D Mumps

   E Hand, foot and mouth disease

1.38   B

Primary varicella zoster infection leads to chickenpox (varicella), which may rarely result in complications including encephalitis and pneumonia. Even when clinical symptoms of chickenpox have resolved, the varicella zoster virus remains dormant in the nervous system of the infected person (virus latency) – in the trigeminal and dorsal root ganglia. In about 10–20% of cases, varicella zoster reactivates later in life to cause a disease known as herpes zoster or shingles.

1.39   D

Mumps is a viral disease of the human species, caused by the mumps virus. Prior to the development of vaccination and the introduction of a vaccine, it was a common childhood disease worldwide, and is still a considerable threat to health in the developing world. Painful swelling of the salivary glands (classically the parotid gland) is the most typical presentation. Painful testicular swelling and rash may also occur. The symptoms are generally not severe in children. In adolescent boys and men, complications such as infertility or subfertility are more common, although still rare in absolute terms.

2
Oral Surgery

2.1 Which one of the following nerves is most likely to be affected in a patient presenting with deviation of the tongue, on protrusion, to the side of a recent submandibular gland excision?

A Accessory

B Facial

C Hypoglossal

D Trigeminal

E Vagus

2.2 Which of the following tumours is the most commonly malignant tumour of the parotid gland?

A Adenocarcinoma

B Adenoid cystic carcinoma

C Mucoepidermoid carcinoma

D Pleomorphic adenoma

E Squamous cell carcinoma

2.3 Which one of the following medications is most likely to complicate the extractions of retained incisor roots?

A Azathioprine

B Allopurinol

C Metformin

D Propranolol

E Zoledronate

2.4 Which one of the following best describes the risk of permanent nerve damage after removal of a mandibular third molar?

A 0.3%

B 3%

C 6%

D 9%

E 12%

2.1   C

Several important nerves travel close to the gland, including the nerve for tongue movement (hypoglossal nerve), the nerve for tongue sensation (lingual nerve) and the branch of the facial nerve responsible for movement of the corner of the lower lip. The risk of damage to either the lingual or the hypoglossal nerve is very minimal, and the damage is almost always temporary. The risk of facial nerve injury leading to permanent paralysis of the lower lip is <1–2%.

2.2   C

A pleomorphic adenoma is the most commonly found benign tumour of the parotid gland; however, the mucoepidermoid carcinoma is the most commonly found malignant tumour of the parotid gland. Squamous cell carcinoma can be found normally as a metastasis from the forehead region.

2.3   E

Zoledronate is a bisphosphonate, and is likely to cause bisphosphonate-induced osteonecrosis of the jaw. Bisphosphonates, when administered intravenously for the treatment of cancer, have been associated with osteonecrosis of the jaw, with the mandible twice as frequently affected as the maxilla, most cases occurring after high-dose intravenous administration used for some cancer patients. Sixty per cent of cases are preceded by a dental surgical procedure, and it has been suggested that bisphosphonate treatment should be postponed until after any dental work to eliminate potential sites of infection.

2.4   B

Inferior alveolar nerve injury related to third molar surgery is reported to occur permanently in up to 3.6% of patients and temporarily in 8% of patients.

Factors associated with inferior alveolar nerve injury include:

- Age
- Difficulty of surgery
- Proximity of inferior alveolar nerve canal.

Renton T. Prevention of iatrogenic inferior alveolar nerve injuries in relation to dental procedures. *Dental Update* 2010;**37**:350–2, 354–6, 358–60.

2.5 Which one of the following is not a complication of removal of mandibular wisdom teeth?

    A   Dry socket

    B   Anaesthesia of the inferior dental nerve

    C   Paraesthesia of the facial nerve

    D   Paraesthesia of the lingual nerve

    E   Trismus

2.6 Which is the correct acronym for a common treatment of a fractured mandible?

    A   OTIF

    B   ORIF

    C   RIMA

    D   LIMA

    E   OSIM

2.7 Which is the resorbable suture of choice when suturing intra-orally after a surgical extraction?

    A   Black silk suture 3/0

    B   Polypropylene 3/0

    C   Vicryl 3/0

    D   Prolene 3/0

    E   Catgut 3/0

2.8 An incisional biopsy is indicated in which one of the following lesions?

    A   Squamous cell carcinoma

    B   Fibroepithelial polyp of the lip

    C   Buccal haemangioma

    D   Palpable submandibular gland lump

    E   Amalgam tattoo

2.5   C

Consent for mandibular wisdom tooth removal should include inferior dental/lingual nerve paraesthesia/anaesthesia, pain, swelling, bruising, need for antibiotics and analgesia. The facial nerve is not involved.

2.6   B

ORIF stands for open reduction and internal fixation. This is one of the most common ways of treating a fractured mandible. It involves an operation to realign and fix the mandible in place, most commonly with plates and monocortical non-compression screws ± intermaxillary fixation. RIMA and LIMA stand for right internal mammary artery and left internal mammary artery, respectively, and are commonly used in coronary artery bypass grafting.

2.7   C

Catgut is a resorbable suture, but it has not been used for years. Its use is now illegal. All the other suture materials apart from Vicryl require removal.

2.8   A

An excisional biopsy is contraindicated in squamous cell carcinoma but is indicated for a fibroepithelial polyp. An amalgam tattoo requires no treatment. Submandibular gland lumps are investigated via fine needle aspiration. A haemangioma should not be biopsied, as it may well bleed dangerously and be life-threatening.

2.9 **After repair of an oroantral fistula, Which one of the following is unnecessary?**

A Analgesia

B Antibiotics

C Ephedrine nasal spray/drops

D Steam inhalations

E Referral to ENT team

2.10 **Which one of the following is not a common sign of a fractured zygoma?**

A Subconjunctival haemorrhage with no visible boundary

B Diplopia

C Paraesthesia of the infra-orbital nerve

D Epistaxis

E Anosmia

2.11 **Which one of the following statements regarding the temporomandibular joint is correct?**

A The disc attaches to the capsule anteriorly

B The articular surface of the disc is made of hyaline cartilage

C The articular surfaces are covered with hyaline cartilage

D The articular surfaces are covered with fibrocartilage

E The middle region of the disc is the most vascular region

2.9 E

A referral to ENT is unnecessary as the treatment is very often successful. All of the other choices are usually prescribed postoperatively.

2.10 E

Anosmia is loss of smell and commonly occurs when the olfactory bulb is damaged. There are many causes of diplopia. The infra-orbital nerve exits from the infra-orbital foramen on the zygoma, and is easily damaged or bruised. Epistaxis occurs when blood leaks from the maxillary antrum.

2.11 D

The articular surfaces of both the disc and the joint are made of fibrocartilage. The most central part of the disc is avascular.

2.12 **Which one of the following statements regarding the temporomandibular joint is incorrect ?**

    A The temporomandibular joint is related to the lateral aspect of the joint

    B The sphenomandibular ligament is an embryological remnant of Meckel's cartilage

    C The sphenomandibular ligament extends from the spine of the sphenoid to the lingula

    D The stylohyoid ligament extends from the tip of the styloid process to the angle of the mandible

    E The stylomandibular ligament is a remnant of the deep cervical fascia as it passes lateral to the parotid gland

2.13 **Which one of the following is not a risk factor for oral cancer?**

    A Smoking

    B Alcohol

    C Previous trauma to the site

    D Social deprivation

    E Betel nut chewing

2.14 **Which one of the following is an indication for extraction of a lower wisdom tooth?**

    A Anterior crowding

    B The tooth is distoangular in position

    C The patient has had two episodes of pericoronitis

    D To 'balance' the extraction of one tooth on one side of the mandible by extracting the wisdom tooth on the other side of the mandible

    E To appease a patient who has atypical facial pain

2.12   E

The stylomandibular ligament is a remnant of the deep cervical fascia as it passes medial to the parotid gland.

2.13   C

The risk factors for oral cancer include smoking, tobacco chewing, snuff, betel nut, alcohol consumption, immunocompromised patients (human immunodeficiency virus (HIV) infection). Trauma is not a risk factor.

2.14   C

A single episode of pericoronitis can be an indication for extraction of a wisdom tooth, however it has to be extremely severe. The recommendation is two episodes of pericoronitis. None of the other are indications for lower wisdom tooth extraction according to the National Institute for Health and Clinical Excellence (NICE) guidelines.

2.15 **Which one of the following statements regarding the submandibular gland is incorrect?**

A   It is the second largest salivary gland

B   It empties via Wharton's duct

C   It has a duct closely related to the lingual nerve

D   It produces entirely serous saliva

E   It is most commonly affected by salivary calculi

2.16 **Xerostomia does not:**

A   Occur after radiotherapy

B   Occur in patients with Sjögren's disease

C   Occur during panic attacks

D   Cause an increase in root caries

E   Occur when taking pilocarpine

2.17 **Which one of the following statements regarding the maxillary sinus is incorrect?**

A   It develops by pneumatisation

B   It is the largest of the paranasal sinuses

C   When fully grown it is pyramidal in shape

D   It is lined by pseudostratified ciliated columnar epithelium

E   It drains via the ostium into the inferior meatus of the nose

2.15 D

The submandibular gland produces mixed saliva. The lingual nerve is very easily damaged during removal of salivary calculi as it loops around Wharton's duct.

2.16 E

Pilocarpine is actually the treatment for xerostomia. Patients with Sjögren's syndrome are prone to dry mouth, dry eyes and dry mucous membranes. Panic attacks lead to dryness of the mouth.

2.17 E

The maxillary sinus drains via the ostium into the middle meatus of the nose. It is small at birth (1 cm) and grows by pneumatisation to become the largest of the paranasal sinuses.

2.18 Which one of the following methods of treatment is inappropriate for the reduction of a fractured mandibular angle in a dentate patient?

A Inter-maxillary fixation (IMF) with a Gunning splint

B IMF using arch bars

C IMF using eyelet wires

D IMF using mini plates and monocortical non-compression screws

E IMF using Leonard's buttons

2.19 What is the most common cause of a fractured mandible?

A Road traffic accidents

B Inter-personal violence

C Sporting injury

D Industrial accidents

E Iatrogenic following wisdom tooth extraction

2.20 What is the correct treatment for an asymptomatic torus palatinus?

A Antibiotics

B Excision

C Incisional biopsy

D Excisional biopsy

E None of the above

2.18 A

IMF using a Gunning splint is a perfectly good treatment for fixation of a fractured mandible, however only in patients who are edentulous. They are splints which are wired to both the mandible and the maxilla and enable IMF to be achieved so that the fracture can be immobilised, and therefore is allowed to heal.

2.19 B

Inter-personal violence is the most common cause of a fractured mandible. Previously road traffic accidents were the major cause, but the advent of the seatbelt laws resulted in a decreased incidence of these fractures from this cause.

2.20 E

No treatment should be prescribed for an asymptomatic torus palatinus. Rarely they have chronic trauma and get secondarily infected, or when dentures are required and it interferes with the design, it needs to be removed.

2.21 **Osteoradionecrosis:**

A Is treated with 100% oxygen

B Commonly affects the maxilla

C Commonly occurs following chemotherapy

D Occurs due to a reduction in vascularity secondary to endarteritis obliterans

E Is the same as focal sclerosing osteomyelitis

2.22 **After extraction of a lower right first molar, how long should you keep the records for?**

A 1 year

B 4 years

C 11 years

D 25 years

E 50 years

2.23 **After the extraction of the lower right first permanent molar; which one of the following conditions would sterilisation of the instruments be achieved?**

A 112 °C for 15 minutes

B 112 °C for 5 minutes

C 121 °C for 15 minutes

D 121 °C for 5 minutes

E 134 °C for 1 minute

2.21   D

Osteoradionecrosis is frequently treated with hyperbaric oxygen, occurs in the mandible, and commonly occurs following radiotherapy. Focal sclerosing osteomyelitis occurs after a low-grade infection, which mainly affects children.

2.22   C

Notes for adult patients should be kept for 11 years. Children's notes should be kept for 11 years or until the patient is 25 years of age, whichever is the longer.

2.23   C

For sterilization to occur at 134 °C it requires the temperature to be maintained for 3 minutes at least. At 121 °C it requires a maintenance of the temperature for 15 minutes for sterilization to occur.

2.24 **Which one of the following drugs is safe to prescribe if the patient has penicillin allergy?**

    A   Augmentin

    B   Ampicillin

    C   Flucloxacillin

    D   Clarithromycin

    E   Cefuroxime

2.25 **What is the name of the instrument shown below?**

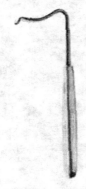

    A   Howarth's periosteal elevator

    B   Bowdler–Henry Rake retractor

    C   Ward's buccal retractor

    D   Laster's retractor

    E   Straight Warwick–James elevator

2.24   D

All of the other drugs are related to penicillin and can cause lethal anaphylaxis if given to those who are allergic to penicillin.

2.25   B

This shows a Bowdler–Henry rake retractor.

2.26 Which tooth would you extract using the forceps shown?

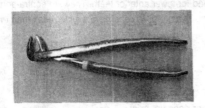

- A Lower left eight
- B Upper left six
- C Lower left two
- D Upper left two
- E Lower right six

2.27 What is the name of the instrument shown below?

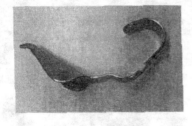 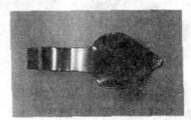

- A Laster's retractor
- B Ward's buccal retractor
- C Howarth's periosteal elevator
- D Bowdler–Henry rake retractor
- E Collins' cheek retractor

2.26 C

These forceps are used for lower anterior teeth. They are contra-angled, which rules out the maxillary teeth. The molar forceps have a wider beak than the anterior teeth forceps.

2.27 A

Collins' cheek retractor does not exist.

2.28 **What would you use the instrument shown in Question 2.27 for?**

    A Lower wisdom tooth extraction

    B Upper wisdom tooth extraction

    C Maxillary advancement osteotomy

    D Sialography

    E Apicectomy

2.29 **Which one of the following statements regarding the muscles of mastication is correct?**

    A The temporalis can be divided into anterior, middle and posterior fibres, all of which carry out the same movements

    B The posterior fibres contribute to the protrusion of the mandible

    C The anterior and middle fibres contribute to the retrusion of the mandible

    D The anterior and middle fibres contribute to the elevation of the mandible

    E The anterior and middle fibres contribute to the protrusion of the mandible

2.30 **Which antibiotic should be prescribed post-operatively, after a surgical extraction?**

    A Clindamycin

    B Metronidazole

    C Amoxicillin

    D Erythromycin

    E Cefuroxime

2.31 **What is the motor nerve supply to the tongue?**

    A Lingual nerve

    B Glossopharyngeal nerve

    C Hypoglossal nerve

    D Vagus nerve

    E Facial nerve

2.28 B

Laster's retractor is used for the retraction of mucoperiosteal flaps to aid visibility during surgical extraction of upper wisdom teeth.

2.29 D

The temporalis has three parts, which produce different movements. The posterior fibres retract the mandible, and the other fibres elevate the mandible.

2.30 B

Metronidazole is the correct antibiotic to be prescribed after surgical extraction. It is effective against anaerobes which are the most common organisms in the mouth.

2.31 C

The hypoglossal nerve is motor to the intrinsic muscles of the tongue, hyoglossus, genioglossus, styloglossus, thyrohyoid and geniohyoid.

2.32 **Which one of the following statements is true?**

    A   The glossopharyngeal nerve serves the posterior third of the tongue for taste only

    B   The glossopharyngeal nerve serves the posterior two-thirds of the tongue for taste only

    C   The glossopharyngeal nerve serves the anterior third of the tongue for taste only

    D   The glossopharyngeal nerve serves the anterior third of the tongue for both taste and sensation

    E   The glossopharyngeal nerve serves the posterior third of the tongue for both taste and sensation

2.33 **Who may be given access to a patient's notes without the patient's permission?**

    A   A patient's employer

    B   A patient's wife or husband

    C   A patient's children

    D   A patient's parents

    E   A defence organisation making allegations of negligence

2.34 **The buccal artery is a direct branch of which artery?**

    A   Mandibular

    B   Maxillary

    C   Facial

    D   External carotid

    E   Internal carotid

2.32 E

Taste sensation to the anterior two-thirds of the tongue is supplied by the chorda tympani via the lingual nerve to the facial nerve. General sensation of the anterior third of the tongue is supplied by the lingual nerve.

2.33 E

A defence organisation may request the records of a patient in regard to a matter of negligence, or you may need to pass records to another healthcare professional, or occasionally you may need to disclose information to a court of law. There should be no other reasons to disclose a patient's records.

2.34 B

The buccal artery is a direct branch of the maxillary artery as are many others including the greater and lesser palatine arteries, the sphenopalatine artery and the middle meningeal artery.

2.35   Which clotting factors does warfarin interfere with?

    A   II, VII, XI, XII

    B   III, V, VII, IX

    C   II, VII, X, XII

    D   II, VII, IX, X

    E   II, III, IX, XI

2.36   The muscle of mastication that helps retract the mandible is:

    A   Temporalis

    B   Masseter

    C   Lateral pterygoid

    D   Medial pterygoid

    E   Buccinator

2.37   A patient has cellulitis involving the tissues of the floor of the mouth and of the sublingual region. The associated swelling happened rapidly and may block the airway. Which eponymous angina does this describe?

    A   Johann's

    B   Ludwig's

    C   Karl's

    D   Jones'

    E   Barnett's

2.35   D

Warfarin interferes with the cyclic process converting the oxidised form of vitamin K to the reduced KH2 form necessary for the production of vitamin K-dependent coagulation factors II, VII, IX and X. Decreased formation of these coagulation factors is responsible for warfarin's anticoagulant effect.

2.36   A

The temporalis is the muscle of mastication that helps in elevation of the mandible. It is large and fan-shaped in appearance and covers the temporal area of the skull.

- Origin and insertion: it originates from the parietal bone of the skull and inserts into the coronoid process of the mandible
- Arterial supply: deep temporal artery
- Nerve supply: trigeminal nerve
- Functions:
  - elevation of the mandible
  - retraction of the mandible
  - crushing of food between the molars

2.37   B

Ludwig's angina is a serious, potentially life-threatening cellulitis infection of the tissues of the floor of the mouth, usually occurring in adults with concomitant dental infections. It is named after the German physician Wilhelm Friedrich von Ludwig who first described this condition in 1836. Ludwig's angina should not be confused with *angina pectoris*, which is also otherwise commonly known as *angina*. The word *angina* comes from the Greek word *ankhon*, meaning strangling, so in this case, Ludwig's angina refers to the feeling of strangling, not the feeling of chest pain, although there may be chest pain in Ludwig's angina if the infection spreads into the retrosternal space.

2.38 Name the instrument shown below

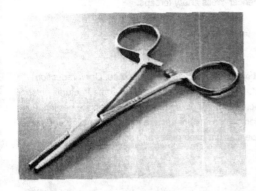

A Mosquito

B Bowdler Henry

C Spencer–Wells

D McIndoe

E Spurr

2.39 What is the acronym used when describing the use of plates and screws to fixate a fractured mandible?

A OBOE

B ORIF

C OTEM

D MIST

E TERM

2.38   C

The picture is of a pair of Spencer–Wells artery forceps.

2.39   B

Open reduction internal fixation (ORIF) is a surgical procedure. *Open reduction* refers to open surgery to set the bones, as is necessary for some fractures. *Internal fixation* refers to fixation of screws and/or plates to enable or facilitate healing. Rigid fixation prevents micro-motion across lines of fracture to enable healing and prevent infection. Some surgeons use titanium bone plates and screws to rigidly fix fractures.

3
Dental Materials

3.1 Which one of the following would be the most appropriate autoclave regimen to adequately sterilise the forceps after the removal of a mandibular molar?

A 110°C for 8 min
B 112°C for 15 min
C 115°C for 8 min
D 115°C for 15 min
E 121°C for 15 min

3.2 You are designing an occlusal rest seat on the mandibular first premolar for a partial cobalt–chrome denture. Which one of the following best describes the optimal depth to which the marginal ridge should be reduced?

A 0.5 mm
B 1.5 mm
C 2.5 mm
D 3.5 mm
E 4.5 mm

3.3 Which of the following metals reduces the amount of creep in an amalgam restoration the most?

A Aluminium
B Copper
C Iron
D Manganese
E Vanadium

3.4 Which of the following is used to increase wetting in dentine bonding systems?

A Acetone
B Carbon tetrachloride
C H_2O
D Methylmethacrylate
D Phosphoric acid

3.1 E

The World Health Organization recommends sterilisation of instruments for 15 min at 121°C.

3.2 B

Marginal ridge must be lowered and rounded 1.0–1.5 mm. The bulk of the metal has to be that thickness to prevent fracture. Any greater depth of preparation causes unnecessary damage to the tooth.

3.3 B

Creep causes protrusion of amalgam out of the cavity; the protruded edges are unsupported and weak, and may be further weakened by corrosion. This leads to fracture, as a result of which there will be a ditch around the margin of amalgam restoration; this will cause a gap and microleakage.

The γ2 phase is primarily responsible for the high value of creep in conventional amalgam, but it is not the only factor involved; high copper amalgam has a lower value of creep because it has a little or no γ2 phase.

3.4 A

Acetone is the best agent for the wetting of dentine. Phosphoric acid is the etchant agent and the derivatives of methylmethacrylate allow a variety of strength in the bond.

3.5 What does an enamel bonding agent consist of?

A   Unfilled resin

B   Filled resin

C   A mixture of resins, acetone and ethanol

D   Wetting agents or resins

E   Prime and bond mixture

3.6 Etched enamel does not need 'wetting' before the enamel bonding agent is applied. Why is 'wetting' not required?

A   Etched enamel has high surface free energy

B   Etched enamel has low surface free energy

C   The enamel bonding agent has a low surface tension

D   The negative charge in the enamel bonding agent is attracted to the positive calcium ions in the etched enamel

E   The negative charge in the enamel bonding agent is attracted to the positive fluoride ions in the etched enamel

3.7 What is the bond strength achievable using enamel bonding agents on etched enamel (1 MPa = 1 kg/mm^2)?

A   0.1 MPa

B   5 MPa

C   30 MPa

D   80 MPa

E   250 MPa

3.5 A

Enamel bonding agents consist of unfilled resin.

3.6 A

The high surface free energy prevents the requirement for 'wetting'. Fluids with a low surface free energy require 'wetting'.

3.7 C

A good bond strength achievable with enamel bonding agents is 30 mPa.

3.8 What is the approximate stress caused by the polymerisation contraction of composite when it is setting?

A 0.1 MPa

B 5 MPa

C 30 MPa

D 80 MPa

E 250 MPa

3.9 Which one of the following is not an advantage of an enamel bonding agent over a dentine bonding agent?

A Decreased marginal leakage

B Better colour stability

C Increased bond strength

D Easier to apply

E Decreased moisture sensitivity

3.10 Which one of the following statements is correct about a dentine primer?

A It etches dentine

B It increases the surface free energy (wets) dentine

C It removes the smear layer

D It bonds to composite

E It conditions the dentine

3.8   B

The approximate stress caused by polymerisation contraction when setting is 5 mPa.

3.9   E

Decreased moisture sensitivity is not an advantage of an enamel bonding agent over a dentine bonding agent. Enamel bonding agents are extremely moisture sensitive.

3.10   B

Dentine primers increase the surface free energy (wet) dentine.

3.11 Which one of the following is true about a dentine 'conditioner'?

    A   It thinly coats collagen fibrils with resin

    B   It thickly coats collagen fibrils with resin

    C   It bonds to composite

    D   It raises the surface free energy of dentine

    E   It removes the smear layer

3.12 The usual enamel bonding agent resin is:

    A   HEMA (hydroxyethyl methacrylate)

    B   Bis-GMA (bisphenol A glycidyl methacrylate)

    C   PENTA (phosphonated penta-acrylate ester)

    D   Dimethylmethacrylate

    E   Polymethylmethacrylate

3.13 The solvent which is used to aid dentine wetting in dentine bonding systems is:

    A   Water

    B   Ethanol or acetone

    C CCl_4 (Carbon tetrachloride)

    D   Ethylene

    E   A low-molecular-weight resin

3.11 E

The main function of the conditioner is to remove the smear layer.

3.12 B

The usual enamel bonding agent resin is Bis-GMA.

3.13 B

The solvent which is used to aid dentine wetting in dentine bonding systems is ethanol or acetone.

3.14 The number of steps in dentine bonding is:

A 1

B 2

C 3

D 4

E Varies

3.15 What is the bond strength between dentine and composite when dentine bonding agents are used?

A 1 MPa

B 5 MPa

C 100 MPa

D 500 MPa

E 1000 MPa

3.16 Which one of the following statements is true about the resin in a dentine bonding agent primer?

A It is hydrophilic

B It is hydrophobic

C It is viscous

D It has a high molecular weight

E It has high surface tension

3.14   E

There are many different systems on the market for dentine bonding, so the number of steps is variable.

3.15   B

The bond strength between dentine and composites when dentine bonding agents are used is 5 MPa.

3.16   B

The resins used in a dentine bonding agent primer are hydrophobic.

3.17 What is the percentage of copper in a high copper dental amalgam alloy?

A 2–12%

B 12–32%

C 32–52%

D 52–70%

E 70+%

3.18 Zinc is often used to improve the properties of amalgam. What happens to a zinc-containing low copper alloy if moisture gets into it?

A The alloy corrodes

B The alloy contracts

C The alloy is reduced

D The alloy expands

E None of the above

3.19 What happens to a zinc-containing high copper alloy if moisture gets into it?

A The alloy corrodes

B The alloy contracts

C The alloy is reduced

D The alloy expands

E None of the above

3.17 B

The percentage of copper in a high copper dental amalgam alloy is between 12% and 32%.

3.18 D

If a zinc-containing low copper alloy is invaded by moisture it expands.

3.19 E

If a zinc-containing high copper alloy is invaded by moisture there is hardly any change.

3.20 Which one of these is a lathe-cut and spherical alloy mixture?

A   Hybrid

B   Admixed

C   Gamma 2

D   Non-gamma 2

E   Gamma 1

3.21 Why is tin added to amalgam?

A   It decreases the reaction rate and gives adequate working time

B   It decreases corrosion

C   It scavenges water molecules

D   It increases filling strength

E   It decreases setting time

3.22 Which one of these chemical compositions is the gamma 1 phase?

A Ag_3Sn

B Ag_2Hg_3

C $AgCu$

D Cu_6Sn_5

E Sn_7Hg

3.20 B

Admixed amalgam contains both lathe-cut and spherical-cut particles.

3.21 A

Tin is added to amalgam to decrease the reaction rate and enables the clinician to have increased working time.

3.22 B

The Ag_3Sn phase is the gamma phase in the silver-tin phase, the Ag_2Hg_3 phase is the gamma phase in the silver-tin phase, and the $Sn_{7-8}Hg$ phase is the gamma phase in the tin-mercury phase. To avoid confusion, the Ag_3Sn is therefore called the gamma phase, the Ag_2Hg_3 the gamma-1 phase, and the Sn_{7-8} the gamma-2 phase.

3.23   Which one of these chemical compositions is the gamma 2 phase?

    A Ag_3Sn

    B Ag_2Hg_3

    C AgCu

    D Cu_6Sn_5

    E Sn_7Hg

3.24   What is the greatest disadvantage of using amalgam in posterior teeth?

    A Mercury toxicity

    B Poor aesthetics

    C Sound tooth tissue requires removal for retention

    D Increased incidence of cusp fracture

    E Decreased lifetime of restoration compared with other materials

3.25   How long does it take for amalgam to form a bond with the tooth?

    A 3 minutes

    B 3 hours

    C 3 days

    D 3 weeks

    E 3 months

3.23 E

Sn_7Hg is the chemical composition in the gamma 2 phase.

3.24 C

As amalgam has no chemical bond to the tooth (unlike composite restorations) it requires mechanical retention, therefore it requires further tooth removal to retain the restoration.

3.25 E

Amalgam takes three months to produce a bond with a tooth.

3.26 Which one of the following statements regarding the properties of casting gold alloys is correct?

    A   The gold content increases on going from soft type I alloy to an extra hard type IV alloy

    B   The corrosion resistance increases on going from a soft type I alloy to an extra hard type IV alloy

    C   The strength increases on going from a soft type I alloy to an extra hard type IV alloy

    D   The ductility increases on going from a soft type I alloy to an extra hard type IV alloy

    E   None of the above statements is correct

3.27 What is the typical particle size in microfilled composite, in micrometres?

    A   0.04

    B   0.4

    C   4

    D   40

    E   400

3.28 What is different about a hybrid composite?

    A   It is a mixture of composite and compomer

    B   It includes a mixture of Bis-GMA and TEG-GMA (triethylene glycol-glycidyl methacrylate)

    C   The filler particles are a combination of silicon dioxide and glass

    D   It is a mixture of composite and glass ionomer

    E   It contains both large and small filler particles

3.26 C

Type I soft casting gold has 85% gold whereas extra hard type IV alloys have only about 65%. This alters the properties of the alloy and the corrosion resistance and the ductility decrease on going from a type I alloy to an extra hard type IV alloy.

3.27 A

The typical particle size of a microfilled composite is 0.04 micrometres.

3.28 E

Answer D defines a compomer. Almost all composites have silicon dioxide and glass filler particles, not just hybrid composites. There is no such mixture as a composite and a compomer.

3.29 **What is the important property of a posterior composite?**

    A   It requires a single cure

    B   It is dual cured

    C   It is very heavily filled

    D   It is very lightly filled

    E   It flows very easily during placement

3.30 **Which one of the following materials should not be used with composites?**

    A   Kalzinol

    B   Zinc phosphate

    C   Vitrebond

    D   Fuji glass ionomer

    E   Poly-F

3.31 **What is the maximum thickness of composite which can be cured by a curing light?**

    A   0.5 mm

    B   1 mm

    C   2 mm

    D   4 mm

    E   6 mm

3.29   C

Single or dual cure is not an important property of a posterior composite. The important property is that the composite is heavily filled so that it can withstand the heavy occlusal forces placed on it. Lightly filled composites and easy flow composites are more commonly used in the anterior region.

3.30   A

Kalzinol prevents bonding of composite to enamel and dentine in a cavity.

3.31   C

The maximum thickness which can be cured is 2 mm. Any thicker than this and your composite will have a 'soggy bottom', and will not be stable as a restoration.

3.32 Which one of the following events does not occur as a result of microleakage at the composite margin?

   A Secondary caries

   B Loss of the restoration

   C Sensitivity

   D Enamel fracture

   E Staining

3.33 Which one of the following is not released from glass ionomer when it sets?

   A Zinc

   B Aluminium

   C Fluoride

   D Calcium

   E Sodium

3.34 When fluoride ions leach out of glass ionomer, what replaces them?

   A Aluminium ions

   B Hydroxyl ions

   C Sodium ions

   D Carbonate ions

   E Silicate ions

3.32 D

The restoration can debond and be lost as a result of microleakage. Also air and fluid leakage can lead to sensitivity, and staining can occur, especially if coloured foods leak around the margins.

3.33 A

Zinc is not released from glass ionomer when it sets. Aluminium, fluoride, calcium and sodium are released during the setting process.

3.34 B

Hydroxyl ions replace the fluoride ions which leach out during the setting process.

3.35 **Which one of the following statements about the curing of composites is true?**

  A   Exposure time of 2–3 seconds is needed for polymerisation with visible light

  B   Before light activation, the base and catalyst are mixed

  C   Lights of both blue and red wavelength are equally effective in polymerisation

  D   Light from an argon laser will activate polymerisation

  E   Light from a lithium laser will activate polymerisation

3.36 **Which one of the following composite fillers is radiopaque?**

  A   Quartz

  B   Lithium aluminium silicate

  C   Colloid silicate

  D   Barium glass

  E   Carbon fibre

3.37 **Which one of the following is the best choice of restorative material to achieve a moderate to high strength restoration that allows fluoride leeching and has good aesthetics?**

  A   Hybrid ionomer

  B   Composite

  C   Compomer

  D   Amalgam

  E   Glass ionomer

3.35   D

Light from an argon laser for usually between 20 and 40 seconds will cure composite.

3.36   D

Barium is a radiopaque material and is used frequently in radiographic investigation. The most common use is in barium enemas. However, this technique is in decline with the increase in computed tomography (CT) scanning.

3.37 A

- **Hybrid ionomers** have been in use for several years, and have found popularity both as restorative materials and as cements for crowns and fixed prostheses. They contain about 80% glass ionomer and 20% resin. The hybrid ionomer releases the fluoride present in the aluminosilicate glass constituent, which is dissolved by the acid present in the mixture. Ongoing research has shown that these restorations release considerable amounts of fluoride during their service in the mouth. The tricure characteristics of hybrid ionomers make them ideally suited for the repair of opaque restorations that have become carious during service. These materials are ideal for the repair of crowns, as well as for repairs in any restorative situation with inadequate light access to allow a light-cured material to cure properly. Hybrid ionomers do not require a bonding agent for retention. They bond to dentine naturally by means of a calcium-carboxylate ion bond. Some manufacturers have suggested using primer before placement of the hybrid ionomer; however, this does not appear to be needed. Ongoing research is showing that the direct contact between the hybrid ionomer and the tooth structure causes high amounts of fluoride to be released into tooth structure. Thus hybrid ionomers are one of the most adequate choices for restoring teeth in patients who have a high caries risk.

- **Compomers** are easier to use than hybrid ionomers, but some of their characteristics are not as desirable as those of hybrid ionomers. Compomers require a bonding agent for adequate retention to dentinal surfaces. The bonding agent reduces the amount of fluoride that can penetrate into the dentine. However, compomers release considerable amounts of fluoride from their external surfaces into the oral environment. These materials are popular for restoration of children's posterior teeth. Because compomers are easy to use, and release fluoride, they are nearly ideal for placement in voids in crown preparations resulting from removal of old silver amalgam or composite restorations (so-called fillers). These materials release less fluoride than hybrid ionomers, but more than typical resin-based composites, most of which release few or no fluoride ions.

- After more than 20 years of use, **conventional glass ionomers** continue to be popular for restoring teeth and for cementing crowns and fixed prostheses. Glass ionomers release considerable amounts of fluoride into tooth structure, as well as into the oral environment. In fact, research has shown them to release more fluoride than any other caries-preventive material. The working characteristics of glass ionomer as a restorative material make it more difficult to use than hybrid ionomer or compomer. Nevertheless, when glass ionomer is used, practitioners can expect it to release considerable amounts of fluoride.

3.38   Which one of the following properties is higher for micro-hybrid composites than for micro-filled composites?

    A   Modulus of elasticity

    B   Water absorption

    C   Thermal expansion

    D   Creep

    E   Polymeric shrinkage

3.39   Regarding adhesion of composite restorations to tooth structure, which one of the following statements is true?

    A   Bonding forms a hybrid layer with enamel

    B   Bonding to enamel is achieved by the application of an acid etchant followed by the application of a bonding agent and then composite resin

    C   The bonding agent forms a micro-mechanical bond with the enamel but a chemical bond with the dentine

    D   Most dentine-bonding agents bond better to a dry surface

    E   Bonding occurs better without rubber dam

3.40   Which one of the following statements applies to packable composites?

    A   Their depth of cure allows bulk polymerisation, which has been shown to be clinically effective

    B   Their wear rate is dissimilar to that of amalgam

    C   They are radiolucent

    D   They have similar or slightly less polymerisation shrinkage than all purpose composites

    E   They exhibit more wear than compomers

3.38   A

An elastic modulus, or modulus of elasticity, is the mathematical description of an object or substance's tendency to deform elastically (ie non-permanently) when a force is applied to it. The elastic modulus of an object is defined as the slope of its stress–strain curve in the elastic deformation region.

3.39   B

B describes the most common pathway for placing a composite.

3.40   A

The packable dental composites can be polymerised in bulk and are clinically very effective.

4
Child Dental Health
and Orthodontics

4.1 How many times a year should a child with high caries risk have fluoride applied to his or her teeth?

    A 1

    B 2

    C 3

    D 4

    E 6

4.2 If a child has an overjet of 11 mm, which category of index of orthodontic treatment need (IOTN) would this demonstrate?

    A 1

    B 3

    C 5

    D 7

    E 9

4.3 A 14-year-old child attends your practice and requests tooth whitening. What should you do?

    A Agree to the treatment because the child is Gillick competent

    B Refuse to treat the child because she is aged 14 years

    C Discuss the request with the parents alone

    D Discuss the request with the parent and child, and obtain permission from both

    E Ask another dentist to witness the child's request and, if he or she is in agreement, proceed with treatment

4.4 Evidence from which one of the following study designs would most support the use of fluoridation in the water supply?

    A Case–control study

    B Cross-sectional study

    C Cohort study

    D Randomised controlled trial

    E Systematic review

4.1 D

Although fluoride is a controversial topic, Newbrun published recommendations suggesting that children of high caries risk require fluoride to be applied topically by a professional four times per year.

Newbrun E. Topical fluorides in caries prevention and management: a North American perspective. *J Dent Educ* 2001;**65**:1078–83.

4.2 C

The British Society of Orthodontics defines the IOTN as follows:

The Dental Health Component (DHC) has five grades:

- *Grade 1* is almost perfection,
- *Grade 2* is for minor irregularities such as:
  - slightly protruding upper front teeth
  - slightly irregular teeth
  - minor reversals of the normal relationship of upper and lower teeth that do not interfere with normal function.
- *Grade 3* is for greater irregularities that normally do not need treatment for health reasons:
  - upper front teeth that protrude <4 mm more than normal
  - reversals of the normal relationship of upper teeth that interfere with normal function only to a minor degree, by <2 mm
  - irregularity of teeth that are <4 mm out of line
  - open bites of <4 mm
  - deep bites with no functional problems.

- *Grade 4* is for more severe degrees of irregularity and these do require treatment for health reasons:

  - upper front teeth that protrude >6 mm

  - reversals of the normal relationship of upper teeth that interfere with normal function >2 mm

  - lower front teeth that protrude in front of the upper by >3.5 mm

  - irregularity of teeth that are >4 mm out of line

  - fewer than the normal number of teeth (missing teeth) where gaps need to be closed

  - open bites of >4 mm

  - deep bites with functional problems

  - more than the normal number of teeth (supernumerary teeth).

- *Grade 5* is for severe dental health problems:

  - when teeth cannot come into the mouth normally because of obstruction by crowding, additional teeth or any other cause

  - a large number of missing teeth

  - upper front teeth that protrude >9 mm

  - lower front teeth that protrude in front of the upper by >3.5 mm and where there are also functional difficulties

  - craniofacial anomalies such as cleft lip and palate.

The aesthetic component

The NHS does realise that some children need orthodontic treatment just because their teeth look really bad. The aesthetic component (AC) is a scale of 10 colour photographs showing different levels of dental attractiveness. The grading is made by the orthodontist matching the patient to these photographs. The photographs were arranged in order by a panel of laypeople.

4.3   D

The child may well be competent to consent to treatment; however, this is an aesthetic treatment, and not one that is medically necessary. In this case, as the child is not an adult, it is appropriate that consent is gained from both parent and child.

4.4   E

For issues of therapy or treatment, the *highest* possible *level of evidence* is a *systematic review* or meta-analysis of randomised controlled trials. Therefore the systematic review provides a higher level of evidence than a randomised controlled trial.

4.5 **Which one of the tables below shows the correct dates of root completion for permanent teeth?**

A

Tooth	Root completion age (years)
Maxillary lateral incisor	8
Maxillary first permanent molar	10–12
Mandibular canine	12–14
Mandibular second permanent molar	17

B

Tooth	Root completion age (years)
Maxillary lateral incisor	13
Maxillary first permanent molar	10–12
Mandibular canine	14–15
Mandibular second permanent molar	12–14

C

Tooth	Root completion age (years)
Maxillary lateral incisor	11
Maxillary first permanent molar	14–15
Mandibular canine	12–14
Mandibular second permanent molar	14–15

D

Tooth	Root completion age (years)
Maxillary lateral incisor	11
Maxillary first permanent molar	9–10
Mandibular canine	12–14
Mandibular second permanent molar	14–15

E

Tooth	Root completion age (years)
Maxillary lateral incisor	9
Maxillary first permanent molar	10–12
Mandibular canine	13–15
Mandibular second permanent molar	18–21

4.5 D

The root completion dates can be worked out from the order of eruption in these four teeth. The order of eruption is maxillary first permanent molar, followed by maxillary lateral incisor, then the mandibular canine then finally the mandibular second permanent molar.

4.6 What is the definition of subluxation?

A The loss of a tooth from the socket which is then replaced within that socket

B The loosening of the tooth within the socket without any displacement

C Injury to the supporting tissues of a tooth without displacement

D Injury to the supporting tissues of a tooth with displacement

E Trauma causing fracture of the alveolar bone leading to displacement

4.6   B

Answer A defines reimplantation, C defines concussion, and the others are not specific definitions.

4.7 What is the recommended dosage of fluoride tablets and drops (mg F/day), related to the concentration of fluoride in the drinking water?

A

Age	< 0.3 ppm F	0.3–0.7 ppm F	> 0.7 ppm F
< 6 months	0	0	0
6 month – 2 years	0.25	0	0
2–4 years	0.5	0.25	0
> 4 years	1.0	0.5	0

B

Age	< 0.3 ppm F	0.3–0.7 ppm F	> 0.7 ppm F
< 6 months	0.5	0.25	0
6 months – 2 years	0.75	0.5	0
2–4 years	1.0	0.75	0.5
> 4 years	2.0	1.0	0.75

C

Age	< 0.3 ppm F	0.3–0.7 ppm F	> 0.7 ppm F
< 6 months	0	0	0
6 months – 2 years	0	0	0
2–4 years	0	0.25	0
> 4 years	1.0	0.5	0

D

Age	< 0.3 ppm F	0.3–0.7 ppm F	> 0.7 ppm F
< 6 months	0	0	0
6 months – 2 years	0	0	0
2–4 years	0.5	0	0
> 4 years	0.4	0.25	0

E

Age	< 0.3 ppm F	0.3–0.7 ppm F	> 0.7 ppm F
< 6 months	0	0	0
6 months – 2 years	1.0	0.5	0.25
2–4 years	2.5	5.0	7.5
> 4 years	10	5	2.5

4.7   A

This is something that needs to be learnt and can be found in the *British National Formulary (BNF)*.

4.8   A Class II division 2 malocclusion as defined by Angle is:

A   The lower arch should be at least one-half cusp width posterior to the upper and the upper central incisors should be proclined

B   The upper arch should be at least one-half cusp width posterior to the upper and the upper central incisors should be retroclined

C   The upper arch should be at least one-half cusp width posterior to the upper and the upper central incisors should be proclined

D   The lower arch should be at least one-half cusp width too far forward to the upper and the upper central incisors should be retroclined

E   The lower arch should be at least one-half cusp width posterior to the upper and the upper central incisors should be retroclined

4.9   Which one of the following may be a sign that a child has been wearing their orthodontic appliance?

A   The acrylic still has a glossy sheen

B   Poor speech

C   The springs are loose at the review appointment

D   The child is having difficulty inserting their appliance

E   There is no change in the occlusion

4.10   A panicking mother informs you that her 3-year-old child's upper central deciduous incisor had avulsed. What advice would you give her?

A   Store the tooth in milk and bring the child to the surgery immediately

B   Store the tooth in cold water and bring the child to the surgery

C   Tell the mother to try to reinsert the tooth into the socket, apply pressure and attend the surgery

D   Attend the surgery immediately with the tooth, but no special precautions for storage of the tooth

E   Store the tooth in chlorhexidine mouthwash and attend the surgery immediately

4.8   E

The starting point of the thought process of elimination should be that Class II division 2 consists of retroclined central incisors. The lower arch is post-normal and therefore this leaves E as the only option.

4.9   C

This is the only sign of use, as the springs would be loose because of the movement of the teeth. The acrylic would be dulled by the saliva in the mouth, the child's speech would have adapted to the appliance, and he or she would be competent at inserting the appliance.

4.10   D

The clue is in the age of the patient. The child is three years old and has only deciduous teeth, which should not be reimplanted. It is prudent to see the child immediately at the practice to check that the entire tooth has avulsed, and to check for any other injuries to the child.

4.11 What is the material of choice for a devitalising pulpotomy?

A Calcium hydroxide

B Formocresol

C Ferric sulphate

D Beechwood creosote

E Tranexamic acid

4.12 A 9-year-old child requires extraction of her upper right first permanent molar under local anaesthesia. Her medical history is unremarkable except that she had rheumatic fever at 3 years of age and a chest infection 4 months ago, which was treated with penicillin. What is the correct precaution for this child?

A No antibiotics required for prophylaxis

B 600 mg clindamycin orally 1 hour pre-operatively

C 750 mg amoxicillin orally 1 hour pre-operatively

D 3 g amoxicillin orally 1 hour pre-operatively

E 3 g amoxicillin intravenously 1 hour pre-operatively

4.13 A 13-year-old child presents with a retained upper left deciduous canine. The successor is not palpable. What would be the most appropriate investigations?

A Orthopantomogram (OPG) and periapical radiograph

B Periapical radiograph

C Vitality test of the deciduous canine

D OPG

E Lateral cephalogram

4.11   C

Formocreosol or Beechwood Creosoate used to be indicated for a non-vital pulpotomy, however there have been concerns about the oncogenic nature of the above treatments. Ferric sulphate is now the treatment of choice. Tranexamic acid is used after extraction in cases where haemostasis has not been achieved.

4.12   A

Pre-operative antibiotic prophylaxis is no longer recommended in this case (NICE, 2008).

4.13   A

This is known as the parallax technique, and enables you to assess whether the missing tooth is placed palatally or buccally. If the tooth is palatally placed it will appear to have moved in the same direction as the X-ray tubehead. If the converse is true then it is placed buccally.

4.14   Which one of the following defines the Frankfort plane?

   A   Distance between the upper and lower incisors in the vertical plane

   B   Line joining porion (superior aspect of external auditory meatus) with orbitale (lowermost point of bony orbit)

   C   Distance between the upper and lower incisors in the horizontal plane

   D   Line joining nasion (most anterior point on fronto-nasal suture) with orbitale (lowermost point of bony orbit)

   E   Line joining porion (superior aspect of external auditory meatus) with nasion (most anterior point on fronto-nasal suture)

4.15   Which one of the following does not cause staining of teeth?

   A   Porphyria

   B   Products of pulpal necrosis

   C   Cefotaxime

   D   Chlorhexidine

   E   Tetracycline

4.16   A patient presents with an increased overjet of 7 mm, an anterior open bite of 5 mm, and a lower left second permanent molar partially erupted and impacted against the first permanent molar. Which Index of Orthodontic Treatment Need (IOTN) category would the patient fall into?

   A   1 (none)

   B   2 (little)

   C   3 (moderate)

   D   4 (great)

   E   5 (very great)

4.14   B

A defines overbite, C defines overjet and the others are false.

4.15   C

Porphyria causes red staining of teeth, products of pulpal necrosis lead to a grey appearance of the enamel, chlorhexidine leads to brown staining and tetracycline leads to blue/brown banding of the teeth.

4.16   D

Having an overjet 6–9 mm, an open bite of greater than 4 mm and partially erupted, impacted teeth places the patient in the IOTN 4 category. Even if you are not entirely familiar with the system, the description tends to suggest that the patient is in great need of treatment.

4.17 Which one of the following tables shows normal measurements on a cephalometric tracing?

A

Measurement	Angle (in degrees)
SNA	81 ± 3
SNB	79 ± 3
ANB	3 ± 2

B

Measurement	Angle (in degrees)
SNA	79 ± 3
SNB	3 ± 3
ANB	81 ±2

C

Measurement	Angle (in degrees)
SNA	81 ± 3
SNB	3 ± 3
ANB	79 ±2

D

Measurement	Angle (in degrees)
SNA	79 ± 3
SNB	81 ± 3
ANB	3 ±2

E

Measurement	Angle (in degrees)
SNA	3 ± 2
SNB	79 ± 3
ANB	81 ±2

4.17 A

These angulations are very important to know as they enable you to correlate your clinical findings with your radiographic findings. This enables you to confirm the classification of your patient skeletally.

4.18 Which one of the following defines the mandibular plane?

A   Porion to orbitale

B   Posterior nasal spine to anterior nasal spine

C   Gonion to menton

D   Porion to menton

E   Gonion to porion

4.19 An anxious mother presents to your surgery with her 4-month-old child who is febrile, has cervical lymphadenopathy, and a combination of vesicles and ulcers on the gingivae and oral mucosa. What is your diagnosis?

A   Teething

B   Dentoalveolar abscess

C   Primary herpetic gingivostomatitis

D   Impetigo

E   Traumatic ulceration

4.20 A child presents with a mid-third root fracture of his upper right permanent central incisor. You choose to splint this tooth, and the mother asks 'For how long will the splint be on the teeth?' You reply:

A   1 week

B   1 month

C   2-3 months

D   6 months

E   1 year

4.18   C

Knowing the anatomical points of a cephalometric tracing are important, and the only two points which are on the mandible are gonion and menton. The gonion is defined as the most posterior inferior point on the angle of the mandible. Menton is defined as the lowermost point on the mandibular symphysis.

4.19   C

The child has lymphadenopathy which rules out A and E. Impetigo presents periorally, not intraorally. The description is of primary herpetic gingivostomatitis, and should be managed with soft diet, fluids and review.

4.20   C

The fracture is unlikely to have calcified by 1 month, and if the splint is left on for more than 3 months the chances of ankylosis are increased.

4.21 Which one of the following statements regarding how deciduous molars differ from permanent molars is correct?

A Deciduous molars have thinner enamel, a less bulbous crown and larger pulp horns than permanent molars

B Deciduous molars have thinner enamel, a more bulbous crown and smaller pulp horns than permanent molars

C Deciduous molars have thinner enamel, a less bulbous crown and smaller pulp horns than permanent molars

D Deciduous molars have thicker enamel, a less bulbous crown and larger pulp horns than permanent molars

E Deciduous molars have thinner enamel, a more bulbous crown and larger pulp horns than permanent molars

4.22 A failure of fusion of which of the following leads to formation of a cleft lip?

A Lateral palatal shelves and the primary nasal process

B Maxillary processes and the median nasal process

C Maxillary processes and the lateral palatal shelves

D Mandibular processes and the maxillary processes

E Lateral palatal shelves and the median nasal processes

4.23 Patients with a cleft palate often have which skeletal relationship?

A Class I

B Class II division 1

C Class II division 2

D Class II division 1 or class II division 2

E Class III

4.21 E

The greater bulbosity of the crown makes it more difficult to place a matrix band on deciduous molars. The pulp horns are larger in deciduous teeth.

4.22 B

A cleft lip is formed because of the failure of fusion of the maxillary and median nasal processes. This is to be differentiated from cleft palate which is formed by the failure of the lateral palatal shelves to rotate downwards and fuse behind the primary palate.

4.23 E

Due to the failure of the maxilla to grow in proportion with the rest of the face, the maxilla is often smaller than the mandible and therefore the patient has a skeletal class III relationship.

4.24 A 15-year-old patient who is still a thumb sucker attends your surgery for an orthodontic assessment. Which malocclusion is she likely to have?

    A   Posterior open bite

    B   Anterior open bite

    C   Increased overbite

    D   Median diastema

    E   Class III skeletal relationship

4.25 Which one of the following is not a good method of child behaviour management?

    A   Behaviour shaping

    B   Desensitisation

    C   Tell, show, do

    D   Positive reinforcement

    E   Sensitisation

4.26 The freeway space is defined as:

    A   The interocclusal clearance when the mandible is in the rest position

    B   The projection of the jaws from beneath the cranial base

    C   The space between the occlusal surfaces of the teeth when the mandible is in a position of habitual posture

    D   The sagittal movement of the mandible during closure from a habitual position to centric occlusion

    E   The position of the mandible when the muscles which are acting on it show minimal activity

4.24   B

Thumb sucking leads to proclination of the upper incisors and retroclination of the lower incisors which can cause a decreased overbite or anterior open bite. The patient may have a median diastema or class III skeletal relationship, but this would not be as a result of the thumb sucking.

4.25   E

The first four are well-recognised behaviour management techniques. Sensitisation is the opposite of what we are trying to achieve.

4.26   A

B defines prognathism, C defines interocclusal clearance, D defines mandibular deviation and E defines the rest position.

4.27 What teeth should a 9-year-old child have in a given quadrant?

   A 12CDE6

   B 1BCDE6

   C 12CDE

   D ABCDE6

   E 1234E6

4.28 What is shown in the figure below?

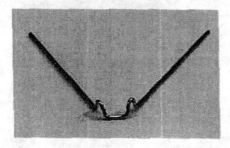

   A A Southend clasp

   B A Roberts retractor

   C An Adams clasp

   D A self-supporting spring

   E A labial bow

4.27   A

Answer B would be more likely for an 8-year-old. Answer D is likely to be a 7-year-old. C and E are not correct.

4.28   C

The image shows an Adams clasp.

4.29 At what age should you try to locate the upper canines?

A 6 years

B 8 years

C 10 years

D 13 years

E 16 years

4.30 Which one of the following is not a cause of a median diastema?

A Normal development

B Microdontia

C Hypodontia

D Lingual frenum

E Midline supernumerary

4.31 Which one of the following is not a part of a removable appliance?

A Active component

B Retention

C Anchorage

D Baseplate

E Bracket

4.29   C

Canines should be located by 10 years of age. It is important to locate them as they are frequently unerupted. This can lead to non-vitality of maxillary lateral and central incisors due to the resorption of their roots. The resorption occurs due to the force of the unerupted canine moving in an incorrect pathway of eruption.

4.30   D

The presence of a lingual frenum has no effect on the positioning of the upper central incisors.

4.31   E

A bracket is a part of a fixed appliance. All the others are important parts of a removable appliance.

4.32   Which one of the following is a side effect of treatment with
       phenytoin, which is commonly prescribed for childhood epilepsy?

    A   Staining of teeth

    B   Gingival hyperplasia

    C   Mental retardation

    D   Taurodontism

    E   Hutchinson's incisors

4.33   What is the angulation of the Frankfort plane?

    A   91°

    B   97°

    C   109°

    D   119°

    E   126°

4.34   When performing inhalational sedation for children, which is the gas
       used?

    A   40% nitrous oxide

    B   100% nitrous oxide

    C   Midazolam

    D   Halothane

    E   Fluothane

4.32   B

Hutchinson's incisors are caused by congenital syphilis. Taurodontism is unrelated to any causative factors, and staining is classically related to tetracycline.

4.33   C

The Frankfort plane is described as the plane through the orbitale and porion. This is meant to approximate the horizontal plane when the head is in the free postural position.

4.34   A

100% nitrous oxide will result in death of the child, midazolam is an intravenous sedation agent, and halothane and Fluothane are general anaesthetic agents.

4.35 In orthodontic treatment planning, which one of the following is incorrect?

    A   Relieve crowding

    B   Correct crossbite

    C   Align arches

    D   Maintain overbite

    E   Maintain overjet

4.36 The overlap of the incisors in the vertical plane is defined as:

    A   Overbite

    B   Overjet

    C   Crossbite

    D   Leeway space

    E   Frankfort plane

4.37 An injury to the supporting tissue of the tooth without displacement of the tooth defines which type of injury?

    A   Concussion

    B   Luxation

    C   Subluxation

    D   Intrusion

    E   Extrusion

4.35   E

When planning orthodontic treatment, one of the aims is to usually reduce or improve the overjet.

4.36   A

The question is asking for the definition of overbite.

4.37   A

Luxation is defined as displacement of the tooth. Subluxation is defined as the loosening of a tooth without displacement. Intrusion is defined as displacement of a tooth into its socket. Extrusion is defined as the partial displacement of a tooth from its socket.

4.38 Which condition is associated with mulberry molars in children?

A Autism

B Down's syndrome

C Osgood syndrome

D Syphilis

E Diabetes mellitus

4.39 When describing cleft lip and palate using Veau's classification, a Veau II involves:

A The soft palate

B The soft and hard palate

C The soft palate, hard palate and the alveolus of one side

D The soft palate, hard palate and the alveolus of both sides

E The Veau classification does not exist

4.40 Which one of the following statements about non-accidental injury is true?

A Usually older children are involved

B Frenal tears are common when a child falls over

C The child and parent's version of events is similar

D It is unusual to find bruises of different vintages on children

E There is often a delay in seeking treatment with these children

4.38 D

A mulberry molar is a tooth with alternating non-anatomical depressions and rounded enamel nodules on its crown surface. It is usually associated with congenital syphilis.

4.39 B

There is no universally accepted classification of clefts, although the most commonly used is the Veau classification, which was described in 1931.

- Veau Class I is an isolated soft palate cleft
- Veau Class II is a hard/soft cleft palate
- Veau Class III is unilateral cleft lip and palate
- Veau Class IV is a bilateral cleft of the lip and palate

Most surgeons describe the defect rather than using the Veau system. For example, a Veau Class III would be described as a unilateral complete cleft of the lip, alveolus, primary and secondary palates.

4.40 E

The features of non-accidental injury are:

- Usually involves younger children
- The injuries do not match the parent's version of events
- Attendance at the hospital or clinic is often delayed
- Bruises appear to be of different vintages
- Frenal tears are an unusual injury
- 50% of children with non-accidental injury have signs of injury on their head or neck

5
Oral Pathology

5.1 A patient who has had bisphosphonate treatment intravenously for multiple myeloma presents with an asymptomatic root-filled, mandibular, first premolar with a periapical radiolucency. How should you proceed?

    A   Extract the tooth under local anaesthetic at the general dental practice

    B   Extract the tooth under local anaesthetic in a hospital setting

    C   Extract the tooth under general anaesthetic in a hospital setting

    D   Re-do the root canal treatment

    E   Observe the tooth over the next 6 months, and take another radiograph

5.2 Which of the following is an odontogenic cyst of developmental origin?

    A   Aneurysmal bone cyst

    B   Epidermoid cyst

    C   Lateral periodontal cyst

    D   Nasopalatine cyst

    E   Residual cyst

5.3 Which one of the following best represents the time (in days) taken for a Vicryl suture to resorb?

    A   5

    B   15

    C   25

    D   35

    E   45

5.4 A 7 year old presents with horizontal linear grooves on the tips of the mandibular and maxillary incisors. What is the most likely cause?

    A   Amelogenesis imperfecta

    B   Childhood illness

    C   Dentinogenesis imperfecta

    D   Hyperfluorosis

    E   Osteogenesis imperfecta

5.1   E

Intravenous bisphosphonate treatment increases the risk of osteochemonecrosis of the jaw post-extraction. The patient is asymptomatic and therefore the most pragmatic thing to do is to observe the patient, and take another radiograph of the tooth in 6 months.

5.2   C

A lateral periodontal cyst is an uncommon type of odontogenic cyst of developmental origin which typically occurs laterally on the root surface of a tooth, representing 0.8–2% of cysts in the jaws. They are frequently located in the mandibular premolar area, followed by the anterior region of the maxilla. It is usually asymptomatic and discovered on a routine radiograph. The involved teeth are usually vital. Although the occurrence of a lateral periodontal cyst is rare, the precision of its diagnosis is necessary so that the correct treatment can be established.

5.3   D

The suture holds its tensile strength for approximately 3–4 weeks in tissue, and is completely absorbed by hydrolysis within 30 days. Vicryl and other polyglycolic acid sutures may also be treated for more rapid breakdown in rapidly healing tissues such as mucous membranes, or impregnated with triclosan to provide antimicrobial protection of the suture line.

5.4   B

Ridging of teeth is frequently caused by childhood illnesses such as measles and chickenpox (varicella). Dentinogenesis and amelogenesis imperfecta cause marked changes in the enamel and the dentine, whereas fluorosis leads to staining of the teeth.

5.5 **Which one of the following statements regarding carcinoma of the lip is true?**

   A   It is commoner on the lower lip

   B   It is often caused by chewing betel nut

   C   It has a worse prognosis than intra-oral carcinoma

   D   It is caused principally by alcohol consumption

   E   It occurs in patients with oral submucous fibrosis

5.6 **Which one of the following is not a microscopic feature of epithelial dysplasia?**

   A   Atypical mitosis

   B   Hyperkeratinisation

   C   Loss of cellular polarity

   D   Altered nuclear/cytoplasmic ratio

   E   Loss or decrease in intercellular adherence

5.7 **Which one of the following statements regarding oral cancer is false?**

   A   It accounts for 2% of all cancers in the UK

   B   It is more common in men

   C   Smoking and alcohol have a synergistic effect

   D   Betel nut is safer than smoked tobacco

   E   It may arise from white patches

5.5 A

Intra-oral carcinoma is principally caused by tobacco products, betel nut, *paan*, and alcohol. Carcinoma of the lip is mainly caused by ultraviolet light, and has a better prognosis because it is more visible, and therefore patients present sooner.

5.6 B

Dysplasia is a term used to describe the histological abnormalities in malignant and premalignant lesions. The abnormal features include unusual mitoses, drop-shaped rete ridges, loss of polarity, and abnormal nuclear cytoplasmic ratio. Hyperkeratinisation is not a feature of dysplasia.

5.7 D

Traditionally oral cancer has been occurring most commonly in males older than 50 years. However, it is being found to occur more often in younger people and its incidence is on the increase, especially in women. Alcohol and smoking do have a synergistic effect, but betel nut is more carcinogenic than smoked tobacco.

5.8 Who proposed in 1889 the acidogenic theory, which is recognised as the correct description of the cause of dental caries?

   A   Miller

   B   Clarke

   C   Jones

   D   Brody

   E   Smith

5.9 Which bacterium is most commonly isolated from root caries?

   A   *Lactobacillus*

   B   *Actinomyces*

   C   *Streptococcus mutans*

   D   *Streptococcus mitior*

   E   *Clostridium*

5.10 Which one of the following epidemiological studies involved the elimination of sucrose and white bread from the diet in an Australian children's home with the subsequent fall in caries in this population during their stay?

   A   Vipeholm study

   B   Hopewood House study

   C   Turku xylitol study

   D   Tristan da Cunha study

   E   Hereditary fructose intolerance study

5.8   A

Miller described the acidogenic theory, which states that acid formed from the fermentation of dietary carbohydrates by oral bacteria leads to the progressive demineralisation of the tooth with subsequent disintegration of the organic matrix.

5.9   B

S. mutans is most frequently isolated from pit and fissure caries, *Lactobacillus* is most commonly isolated from the advancing edge of the carious process in dentine and *Actinomyces* is most commonly isolated from root caries.

5.10   B

In Tristan da Cunha there was low caries incidence until the Americans arrived during the war bringing refined carbohydrates with them, and afterwards the caries rate soared. In the Hopewood House study, the children demonstrated a higher caries rate before and after being in the children's home. The Turku xylitol study showed a 90% caries decrease when xylitol was substituted for sucrose.

5.11   **Which one of the following histopathological zones is the advancing edge of caries in enamel?**

   A   Zone of sclerosis

   B   Translucent zone

   C   Surface zone

   D   Dark zone

   E   Zone of destruction

5.12   **Which one of the following histopathological zones is the advancing edge of the carious lesion in dentine?**

   A   Zone of sclerosis

   B   Dark zone

   C   Surface zone

   D   Zone of demineralisation

   E   Zone of destruction

5.13   **What is chronic hyperplastic pulpitis more commonly known as?**

   A   Acute pulpitis

   B   Pulp polyp

   C   Chronic pulpitis

   D   Acute periapical periodontitis

   E   Chronic periapical periodontitis

5.11 B

See explanation below.

5.12 A

The four zones of dentine caries in order from the advancing edge are:

1. Zone of sclerosis

2. Zone of demineralisation

3. Zone of bacterial invasion

4. Zone of destruction

For enamel the four zones in order from the advancing edge are:

1. Translucent zone

2. Dark zone

3. Body of lesion

4. Surface zone

5.13 B

Clinically a pulp polyp has the appearance of a bright red or pink soft tissue mass within a large carious cavity.

5.14 Which one of the following is a non-odontogenic cyst?

   A   Odontogenic keratocyst

   B   Dentigerous cyst

   C   Eruption cyst

   D   Radicular cyst

   E   Nasopalatine cyst

5.15 Which one of the following cysts is an inflammatory odontogenic cyst?

   A   Odontogenic keratocyst

   B   Dentigerous cyst

   C   Eruption cyst

   D   Radicular cyst

   E   Gingival cyst

5.16 Which one of the following cysts is derived from the root sheath of Hertwig and has the rests of Malassez as an epithelial residue?

   A   Odontogenic keratocyst

   B   Dentigerous cyst

   C   Eruption cyst

   D   Radicular cyst

   E   Gingival cyst

5.14   E

All the other cysts are odontogenic in origin and have an epithelial residue which occurs as the glands of Serres, reduced enamel epithelium or rests of Malassez. The nasopalatine cyst is a heart shaped or ovoid cyst which forms from the remnants of the nasopalatine canal, and is lined by stratified squamous epithelium or pseudostratified squamous epithelium.

5.15   D

All of the other cysts are developmental cysts. There are three types of radicular cyst: apical periodontal cyst (75%), lateral periodontal cyst (5%) and residual cyst (20%). They are the most common type of odontogenic cyst and are responsible for 75% of odontogenic cysts.

5.16   D

The dental lamina is responsible for the production of odontogenic keratocysts and its epithelial residue is the glands of Serres. The enamel organ is responsible for the production of both dentigerous cysts and eruption cysts, and their epithelial residue occurs as the reduced enamel epithelium. Radicular cysts are derived from the root sheath of Hertwig and have the rests of Malassez as the epithelial residue.

5.17 **Where are you most likely to find a radicular cyst?**

 A Maxillary central incisor region

 B Mandibular central incisor region

 C Mandibular premolar region

 D Maxillary premolar region

 E Mandibular third molar region

5.18 **Which one of the following cysts is most likely to recur?**

 A Odontogenic keratocyst

 B Dentigerous cyst

 C Eruption cyst

 D Radicular cyst

 E Gingival cyst

5.19 **Which one of the following non-odontogenic cysts is typically found as a firm mass 2–4 cm in diameter, mostly below the level of the hyoid, occasionally gets infected, and is developmentally related to the foramen caecum?**

 A Lymphoepithelial cyst

 B Nasopalatine cyst

 C Nasoalveolar cyst

 D Thyroglossal duct cyst

 E Dermoid cyst

5.17 A

The maxillary central incisors are responsible for 37% of all radicular cysts. They are frequently traumatised and often occur as asymptomatically non-vital teeth. The radicular cyst is often found as an incidental finding on a radiograph.

5.18 A

Odontogenic keratocysts frequently recur and require close monitoring.

5.19 D

The thyroglossal duct cyst is a remnant of the process of descent of the thyroid gland. It is often found in adolescents and requires excision of part of the hyoid bone as well to prevent recurrence. The function of the thyroid gland is assessed. This can be done by measuring the thyroxine (T4) levels of the patient.

5.20 Which one of the following is not a physical cause of non-carious tooth surface loss?

    A Fracture

    B Attrition

    C Abrasion

    D Vomiting

    E Iatrogenic

5.21 Which one of the following is not a cause of tooth surface loss on the palatal surfaces of maxillary central incisors?

    A Chemotherapy

    B Oesophageal reflux

    C Anorexia

    D Bulimia

    E Pregnancy

5.22 Which one of the following statements regarding acute osteomyelitis is true?

    A It affects the maxilla more than the mandible

    B It always causes paraesthesia of the inferior dental nerve in the mandible

    C It will not be apparent on radiographs for a month

    D It will usually cause sharp shooting pain

    E It may cause the loosening of teeth

5.20   D

Vomiting is a common cause of chemical tooth surface loss. It is the low pH of the vomit that frequently causes the palatal tooth surface loss. All of the others are physical causes of tooth surface loss.

5.21   C

Anorexia involves the reduction in calorific intake to reduce weight gain. Bulimia is the act of ingesting food and then regurgitating it to prevent weight gain. Chemotherapy causes hyperemesis, and this can be quite marked. Oesophageal reflux causes the reflux of acidic stomach contents into the mouth leading to erosion. Pregnancy causes hyperemesis gravidarum in the first trimester which settles normally by the second trimester, but can be present throughout pregnancy.

5.22   E

Osteomyelitis most frequently occurs in the mandible. The pain most commonly associated with osteomyelitis is a severe throbbing pain. It may cause the loosening of teeth, but does not always cause the paraesthesia of the inferior dental nerve when associated with the mandible.

5.23   Regarding Paget's disease which one of the following statements is false?

A   Hypercementosis occurs, leading to ankylosis and difficult extractions

B   Patients with Paget's disease are liable to get post-extraction osteomyelitis

C   Patients with Paget's disease have problems with post-extraction haemorrhage

D   Patients with Paget's disease can have facial nerve paralysis

E   The mandible is more frequently affected than the maxilla in Paget's disease

5.24   What is the most common age of presentation of a giant cell granuloma?

A   Under 5 years

B   10–25 years

C   30–40 years

D   45–65 years

E   65+ years

5.25   Which one of the following statements regarding hairy leukoplakia is true?

A   It only ever occurs in patients with HIV infection

B   It is caused by *Candida*

C   It commonly affects the dorsal surface of the tongue

D   It is a premalignant lesion

E   It has koilocyte-like cells in the prickle cell layer

5.23 E

In Paget's disease the maxilla is more frequently affected than the mandible. This disease was first described by Sir James Paget in 1877, and is a disorder of bone turnover. It occurs in males over the age of 40, and is most common in weight-bearing bones of the axial skeleton such as the sacrum, vertebrae, femur and skull. The patients have bony pain, and the disorder causes compression of nerves leading to paralysis. There is spacing of teeth, and hats and dentures become ill fitting.

5.24 B

Giant cell granulomas occur more frequently in the mandible than in the maxilla, often in the most anterior part of the jaws. They present as a well-defined radiolucent area with thinning and often expansion of the cortex. They may be multi-locular, and involved teeth may be displaced and roots may be resorbed. They heal readily after curettage and are histologically identical to lesions of hyperparathyroidism.

5.25 E

Hairy leukoplakia can occur in patients who are immunocompromised, and is often secondarily infected with Candida. It is not a premalignant lesion.

5.26 Which one of the following statements regarding salivary calculi is true?

    A They may be asymptomatic

    B They are always visible on a lower occlusal radiograph

    C They most frequently occur in the parotid gland

    D They most frequently occur in the sublingual gland

    E They are a common cause of xerostomia

5.27 Which one of the following statements regarding salivary gland tumours is true?

    A Adenoid cystic carcinomas have a good prognosis

    B Acinic cell carcinomas spread perineurally

    C Mucoepidermoid carcinomas histologically have a 'Swiss cheese appearance'

    D Pleomorphic adenomas usually undergo malignant change

    E Pleomorphic adenomas contain fibrous, elastic and myxoid tissue

5.28 Which one of the following statements regarding fibrous dysplasia is true?

    A It is commoner in males

    B It affects the maxilla more than the mandible

    C It is very painful

    D Histologically there is resorption and deposition of bone

    E It commonly occurs in patients around 40 years of age

5.26 A

Salivary gland calculi frequently occur in the submandibular gland. They do not lead to xerostomia, as the parotid gland produces the greatest amount of saliva. These calculi may be seen on plain film radiographs, but sialography may be required to visualise them.

5.27 E

Adenoid cystic carcinomas have a very poor prognosis, spread perineurally and have a 'Swiss cheese' appearance. A small proportion of pleomorphic adenomas (2%) undergo malignant change, but these adenomas contain a variety of tissues, including fibrous, elastic and myxoid tissue.

5.28 B

Fibrous dysplasia is a disease which occurs in women more than men and presents in people younger than 20 years. It is infrequently painful and involves the replacement of bone by fibrous tissue.

5.29 Which one of the following statements regarding osteosarcoma is false?

A   It is a complication of Paget's disease

B   It occurs in men more frequently than women

C   It occurs more commonly in the maxilla than the mandible

D   Patients frequently present between the ages of 30 and 40 years

E   Patients frequently present with paraesthesia

5.30 Which one of the following statements regarding odontomes is true?

A   They are hamartomas

B   They present at the age of 30 years

C   They can undergo a malignant transformation

D   They are frequently present in the anterior mandible

E   The lesion is composed of cementum embedded in fibrous tissue and a surrounding capsule

5.31 Which one of the following conditions is associated with anti-basement membrane auto-antibodies?

A   Erythema multiforme

B   Stevens–Johnson syndrome

C   Pemphigoid

D   Pemphigus

E   Herpes zoster

5.29 C

Osteosarcoma is an infrequent complication of Paget's disease, and occurs in men between the age of 30 and 40 years. It affects the mandible more frequently than the maxilla, and often the presenting complaint is a paraesthesia.

5.30 A

Odontomes usually present between the ages of 10 and 20 years of age, and are benign. They commonly present in the anterior maxilla and the posterior mandible. The lesion is composed of pulp, dentine, enamel and cementum.

5.31 C

Pemphigoid is a subepithelial vesiculo-bullous disorder, which occurs in women over the age of 60. It is characterised by tough bullae, which last for 2–3 days before bursting. It can involve the skin, conjunctiva, nasal and laryngeal regions. It also heals with scarring.

5.32 Which one of the following prenatal/neonatal problems does not affect the dentition?

    A Syphilis

    B Rubella

    C Hypocalcaemia

    D Haemolytic disease of the newborn

    E Zoster

5.33 Which one of the following teeth is most commonly congenitally absent (barring wisdom teeth)?

    A Maxillary central incisor

    B Maxillary lateral incisor

    C Maxillary first premolar

    D Maxillary second premolar

    E Mandibular second premolar

5.34 How many days after fertilisation does the dental lamina develop?

    A 23 days

    B 37 days

    C 51 days

    D 65 days

    E 79 days

5.32   E

All of the other disorders lead to either hypomineralisation of the dentition or a developmental anomaly.

5.33   E

Of people who have a congenitally absent tooth, 40.9% are missing a mandibular second premolar, 23.5% are missing a maxillary lateral incisor, and 20.9% are missing a maxillary second premolar.

5.34   B

The dental lamina develops 37 days after fertilisation, and from this the tooth buds develop.

5.35   What is the typical location of a mesiodens?

A   Between the maxillary central incisors

B   Between the mandibular central incisors

C   Associated with the maxillary canines

D   Associated with the mandibular premolars

E   Associated with the mandibular third molars

5.36   Which one of the following is not an acquired white spot lesion?

A   Keratosis traumatica

B   Smoker's keratosis

C   Hairy leukoplakia

D   Oral candidiasis

E   White sponge naevus

5.35   A

Mesiodentes are the most common supernumerary teeth, occurring in 0.15–1.9% of the population. Mesiodentes can cause delayed or ectopic eruption of the permanent incisors.

5.36   E

White sponge naevus, also known as Cannon's disease or hereditary leukokeratosis of mucosa, appears to follow a hereditary pattern as an autosomal dominant trait. Although it is congenital in most cases, it can develop in childhood or adolescence. It presents in the mouth, most frequently as a thick bilateral white plaque with a spongy texture, usually on the buccal mucosa, but sometimes on the labial mucosa, alveolar ridge or floor of the mouth. The gingival margin and dorsum of the tongue are almost never affected. Although this condition is perfectly benign, it is often mistaken for leukoplakia. There is no treatment, but because there are no serious clinical complications, the prognosis is excellent.

5.37 A pathology report comes back with the following: subepithelial band-like lymphocytic infiltrate with the presence of Civatte bodies and immunoglobulin deposition. This report is describing:

A Squamous cell carcinoma

B White sponge naevus

C Lichen planus

D Rheumatoid arthritis

E Sjögren's disease

5.38 Which one of the following is a mesenchymal odontogenic tumour?

A Ameloblastoma

B Odontogenic fibroma

C Squamous odontogenic tumour

D Calcifying epithelial odontogenic tumour

E Adenomatoid odontogenic tumour

5.37 C

The cause of lichen planus is not known. It is not contagious and does not involve any known pathogen. Some lichen planus-type rashes (known as lichenoid reactions) occur as allergic reactions to medications for high blood pressure, heart disease and arthritis. These lichenoid reactions are referred to as lichenoid mucositis (of the mucosa) or dermatitis (of the skin). Lichen planus has been reported as a complication of chronic hepatitis C virus infection and can be a sign of chronic graft-versus-host disease of the skin. It has been suggested that true lichen planus may respond to stress, where lesions may present on the mucosa or skin during times of stress in those with the disease. Lichen planus affects women more than men (in a ratio of 3:2), and occurs most often in middle-aged adults. Lichen planus in children is rare.

5.38 B

- Mesenchymal odontogenic tumours: odontogenic myxoma, odontogenic fibroma, cementoblastoma, cementifying fibroma

- Epithelial odontogenic tumours: ameloblastoma, squamous odontogenic tumour, calcifying epithelial odontogenic tumour, adenomatoid odontogenic tumour

5.39 Which type of collagen makes up the periodontal ligament?

    A I

    B II

    C III

    D IV

    E V

5.40 Pressure on a tooth root stimulates:

    A Growth

    B Osteoblast activity

    C Osteoclast activity

    D Transforming growth factor release

    E Nothing

5.39 A

Collagen type	Description	Associated conditions
I	This is the most abundant collagen in the human body. It is present in scar tissue, the end product when tissue heals by repair. It is found in tendons, skin, artery walls, the endomysium of myofibrils, fibrocartilage, and the organic part of bones and teeth	Osteogenesis imperfecta, Ehlers–Danlos syndrome
II	Hyaline cartilage, makes up 50% of all cartilage protein. Vitreous humour of the eye	Collagenopathy types II and XI
III	This is the collagen of granulation tissue, and is produced quickly by young fibroblasts before the tougher type I collagen is synthesised. It forms the reticular fibres. Also found in artery walls, skin, intestines and the uterus	Ehlers–Danlos syndrome
IV	This is found in the basal lamina and the eye lens. It also serves as part of the filtration system in capillaries and the glomeruli of nephrons in the kidney	Alport syndrome
V	Mostly occurs in interstitial tissue, associated with type I and the placenta	Ehlers–Danlos syndrome

5.40 C

This is the basic principle of root resorption. The pressure stimulates osteoclast activity, which leads to resorption.

6

Periodontics

6.1   A cohort study was performed to see the outcomes of two different periodontal interventions. What level of evidence would apply to this study?

   A   Level Ia

   B   Level IIb

   C   Level IIIb

   D   Level IVa

   E   Level V

6.2   Which one of the following would be the most appropriate way to clear a periodontal probe of potential prions found in a patient with Creutzfeldt–Jakob disease?

   A   Gamma radiation

   B   Incineration

   C   Soap and water

   D   Sodium hypochlorite

   E   Vacuum autoclave

6.1 B

The most recent table of the Oxford levels of evidence is:

Grade of recommendation	Level of evidence	Type of study
A	1a	Systematic review of (homogeneous) randomised controlled trials
	1b	Individual randomised controlled trials (with narrow confidence intervals)
B	2a	Systematic review of (homogeneous) cohort studies of 'exposed' and 'unexposed' individuals
	2b	Individual cohort study/low-quality randomised controlled trials
	3a	Systematic review of (homogeneous) case–control studies
	3b	Individual case–control studies
C	4	Case studies, low-quality cohort or case–control studies
D	5	Expert opinions based on non-systematic reviews of results or mechanistic studies

6.2 B

Prions are highly resistant to disinfectants, heat, ultraviolet radiation, ionising radiation and formalin. However, prions can be deactivated by heat, chemicals, and a combination of heat, chemicals, pressure and time.

Prions can be destroyed through incineration provided that the incinerator can maintain a temperature of 900°F for 4 hours.

6.3   After establishing drainage, which one of the following is the most
        appropriate first-line antimicrobial for a patient with a lateral
        periodontal abscess, lymphadenopathy and pyrexia?

        A   Amoxicillin

        B   Co-amoxiclav

        C   Chloramphenicol

        D   Erythromycin

        E   Metronidazole

6.4   A 4-year-old child presents with spontaneous bleeding of the
        gingivae. What is the likely diagnosis?

        A   Gingivitis

        B   Gingival hyperplasia

        C   Leukaemia

        D   Lymphoma

        E   Vitamin E deficiency

6.5   Which one of the following statements best describes the diagnosis
        of peri-implantitis?

        A   Bleeding on probing has a low sensitivity and low specificity

        B   Implant mobility has high sensitivity and high specificity

        C   Probing depth has a low sensitivity and high specificity

        D   Pus expelled on digital pressure has high sensitivity and high specificity

        E   Radiographic bone loss has a high sensitivity and low specificity

6.3 E

Metronidazole is a core antibiotic for the treatment of anaerobic infections. Its mechanism of action is not entirely clear, but it is thought that the active metabolite interferes with DNA synthesis.

Metronidazole is active against most anaerobic protozoa including *Giardia lamblia*, *Trichomonas vaginalis*, *Entamoeba histolytica* and *Blastocystis hominis*. Gram-negative anaerobic bacteria, such as those belonging to the *Bacteroides fragilis* group and Gram-positive anaerobic bacteria such as *Peptostreptococcus* and *Clostridium* species, are also usually sensitive to metronidazole.

6.4 C

Presentation is highly variable, depending on the child's age and the extent of leukaemic infiltration of the bone marrow and other sites, as well as cytokine systemic effects:

- The classic signs of anaemia, thrombocytopenia, hepatosplenomegaly or lymphadenopathy are highly suspicious of leukaemia, but initial symptoms are often non-specific and vague and very similar to common, self-limiting, viral illnesses.

- The symptoms and signs listed above are common manifestations of the condition. There is no good evidence base to allow rational decision-making in primary care between phlebotomy and 'wait-and-see' approaches when symptoms are more vague. Where symptoms are prolonged, particularly troublesome or present atypically compared with more common illnesses in children, it may be wise to conduct initial investigations.

6.5 D

Microbiological diagnostics are of high prognostic value and thus comprise an essential support for the choice of appropriate therapy. The microbiological method of determination must be reproducible, demonstrate a high level of specificity and sensitivity, and above all facilitate precise quantification of bacteria in order to supply useful and evaluable information for periodontal treatment. Pus expelled by digital pressure has a high sensitivity and specificity.

6.6 Which one of the following bacterial species is not associated with adult periodontitis?

A *Fusobacterium nucleatum*

B *Bacteroides forsythus*

C *Porphyromonas gingivalis*

D *Shigella sonnei*

E *Prevotella intermedia*

6.7 When looking at the notes of a patient, you see annotation for a Basic Periodontal Examination (BPE). What does a score of 3 mean on this particular index?

A Gingival bleeding, no overhangs or calculus, pockets > 3.5 mm

B Pockets within colour-coded area, 4.5–6.5 mm

C Colour-coded area disappears, pockets > 5.5 mm

D Pockets within colour-coded area, 3.5–5.5 mm

E Colour-coded area disappears, pockets > 5.5 mm

6.8 Which one of the following statements regarding acute necrotising ulcerative gingivitis (ANUG) is true?

A It is caused by Gram-positive anaerobic bacteria

B It is characterised by chronic onset

C It affects non-smokers more than smokers

D It is caused by acid fast bacilli

E It is characterised by interproximal necrosis

6.6   D

All of the bacteria in the list are responsible for adult periodontitis except *S. sonnei*, which is responsible for acute diarrhoea.

6.7   D

The WHO probe is used for carrying out BPE. The index is shown below.

Score	Disease
0	No disease
1	Gingival bleeding, no overhangs or calculus, pockets < 3.5 mm
2	No pockets > 3.5 mm, no supragingival calculus or subgingival overhangs present
3	Pockets within the colour-coded area, 3.5–5.5 mm
4	Colour-coded area disappears, pockets > 5.5 mm

6.8   E

ANUG is caused by Gram-negative aerobic bacteria, usually in the mandible, has a very distinctive smell (fetor oris) and is more common in smokers and those with poor oral hygiene.

6.9   Correct treatment of a patient with ANUG is:

A   20% chlorhexidine mouthwashes twice daily

B   Amoxicillin 500 mg three times daily for 5 days and 20% chlorhexidine mouth washes twice daily

C   Erythromycin 250 mg four times daily for 5 days and 20% chlorhexidine mouthwashes twice daily

D   Scaling and oral hygiene instruction

E   Metronidazole 400 mg three times daily for 5 days and hydrogen peroxide mouthwash twice daily

6.10   Which one of the following statements about tooth mobility is incorrect?

A   Movement of a crown of the tooth in the horizontal plane of less than 0.2 mm is considered normal

B   Grade 1 means movement of the crown of a tooth in the horizontal plane is 0.2–1 mm

C   Grade 2 means movement of the crown of a tooth in the horizontal plane is greater than 1 mm

D   Grade 3 means movement of the crown of a tooth in the horizontal plane is greater than 3 mm

E   Grade 3 means movement of the crown of a tooth in the vertical plane

6.11   Which one of the following clinical conditions predisposes patients with impaired/defective neutrophil function to severe periodontitis?

A   Patterson–Brown–Kelly syndrome

B   Chediak–Higashi disease

C   Hypothyroidism

D   Hyperthyroidism

E   Gardner's syndrome

6.9 E

ANUG is a very painful condition. The most efficacious mouthwash is hydrogen peroxide, and the bacterial component is treated with metronidazole. Amoxicillin and erythromycin would be ineffective in treatment of this condition.

6.10 D

Tooth mobility is graded as shown in the table below.

Grade	Description
1	Movement of the crown of a tooth in the horizontal plane is 0.2–1 mm
2	Movement of the crown of a tooth in the horizontal plane is greater than 1 mm
3	Movement of the crown of a tooth in the vertical plane

6.11 B

None of the others are relevant to periodontal disease.

6.12 Which one of the following is associated with abnormal collagen formation leading to periodontal disease?

    A Type 1 diabetes mellitus

    B Papillon–Lefèvre syndrome

    C Hypophosphatasia

    D Type 2 diabetes mellitus

    E Hyperphosphatasia

6.13 What is the name of the probe shown in the figure?

    A Briault's

    B Community Periodontal Index of Treatment Needs (CPITN)

    C World Health Organization (WHO)

    D Williams'

    E Florida

6.12   C

Hypophosphatasia, as well as Ehlers–Danlos syndrome are associated with abnormal collagen formation and periodontal disease. Papillon–Lefèvre syndrome is associated with abnormal neutrophil function, which leads to periodontal disease.

6.13   D

The probe shown is the Williams' probe, which has 1 mm increments for accurate measurement of the pocket depth.

6.14 In juvenile periodontitis, which bacterium is the recognised aetiological agent?

A *Porphyromonas gingivalis*

B *Prevotella intermedia*

C *Actinobacillus actinomycetemcomitans*

D *Borrelia burgdorferi*

E *Fusobacterium intermedium*

6.15 Which teeth are most commonly affected in juvenile periodontitis?

A Incisors and first permanent molars

B Incisors and canines

C Canines and premolars

D Premolars and first permanent molars

E Canines and first permanent molars

6.16 For which teeth/surfaces would you use a Gracey no 1 or no 2 curette when scaling?

A All teeth

B All surfaces of anterior teeth

C Mesial surfaces of anterior teeth

D All surfaces of posterior teeth

E Mesial surfaces of posterior teeth

6.14 C

A. actinomycetemcomitans is a capnophilic, non-motile rod that possesses a potent leucotoxin, which causes lysis of polymorphonuclear leucocytes.

6.15 A

As these are the first teeth to erupt, they seem to be the teeth which are affected most by juvenile periodontitis.

6.16 B

A Gracey no 1 or no 2 is ideally shaped to facilitate scaling of all surfaces of anterior teeth.

6.17 What pressure should be used when probing for BPE?

 A 5 g

 B 25 g

 C 75 g

 D 150 g

 E 500 g

6.18 Which one of the following statements regarding dental calculus is false?

 A It is mineralised dental plaque

 B It is composed of hydroxyapatite

 C It is the primary cause of periodontitis

 D The outer surface remains covered by a layer of plaque

 E It forms when plaque is mineralised from calcium and phosphate ions

6.17   B

This is the level of force prescribed by the World Health Organization.

6.18   C

The primary cause of periodontitis is plaque, not calculus.

6.19 Match the names of the instruments with the letters underneath them in the figure below

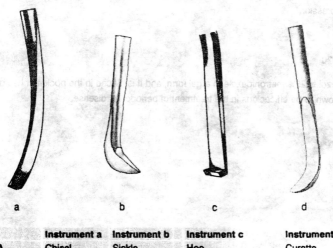

	Instrument a	Instrument b	Instrument c	Instrument d
A	Chisel	Sickle	Hoe	Curette
B	Sickle	Hoe	Chisel	Curette
C	Curette	Hoe	Sickle	Chisel
D	Sickle	Hoe	Curette	Chisel
E	Chisel	Curette	Hoe	Sickle

6.20 What is the active component of Elyzol, a topical antimicrobial placed in deep periodontal pockets?

    A   Tetracycline

    B   Amoxicillin

    C   Clindamycin

    D   Erythromycin

    E   Metronidazole

6.19 A

It is important to know the names of instruments. If you are passed an instrument in a pass/fail viva and you don't know its correct name it doesn't create a very good impression.

6.20 E

Elyzol is 25% metronidazole in a gel form, and it is placed in the pocket. It has been shown to be efficacious in the treatment of periodontal disease.

6.21 After a course of periodontal treatment, how long should you wait to perform a six-point pocket examination to see if there has been any improvement?

    A   Immediately after treatment has finished

    B   1 week

    C   1 month

    D   3 months

    E   6 months

6.22 Which one of the following drugs does not cause gingival hyperplasia?

    A   Ciclosporin

    B   Phenytoin

    C   Phenobarbital

    D   Nifedipine

    E   Diphenylhydantoin (Dilantin)

6.21 D

It takes at least 2 months for healing in the periodontal pocket to occur. Therefore 3 months would be the ideal length of time to wait before performing a six-point pocket chart.

6.22 C

Ciclosporin is an immunosuppressant, phenytoin and Dilantin are anti-epileptics and nifedipine is a calcium channel blocker. They all cause gingival hyperplasia. Phenobarbital does not.

6.23 What procedure is shown in the diagram?

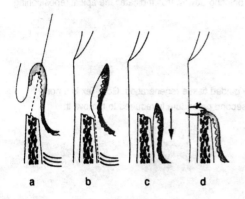

a   b   c   d

- A Modified Widman's flap
- B Simple gingivectomy
- C Apically repositioned flap
- D Coronally repositioned flap
- E Widman's flap

6.24 Which one of the following is not used in guided tissue regeneration?

- A Gore-Tex
- B Autogenous gingival graft
- C Cellulose barrier membrane
- D Collagen barrier membrane
- E Silica

6.23 C

The diagram with the arrow pointing downwards indicates the apical repositioning of the flap.

6.24 E

Silicone not silica is used in guided tissue regeneration. Gore-Tex is a non-resorbable material, and a second procedure is required to remove it.

6.25 If a patient has a BPE score of 2, what is the correct course of treatment?

A   Nothing

B   Oral hygiene instruction (OHI)

C   OHI and scaling

D   OHI, scaling and correction of any iatrogenic factors

E   OHI, scaling and root planing

6.26 A lesion is described as a small apostrophe-shaped or slit-like fissure of the gingivae extending from the gingival margin to a depth of up to 5 to 6 cm. This lesion is normally found between the mandibular central incisors. What is this lesion?

A   McCall's festoon

B   Stillman's cleft

C   O'Leary's cleft

D   Williams' festoon

E   Barnes' festoon

6.25 D

By definition, the score of 2 means that the particular sextant has no pockets of greater than 3.5 mm, and no subgingival calculus or subgingival overhangs are present. Therefore root planing is not indicated.

6.26 B

Stillman's cleft.

6.27   Interleukins (ILs) are important in the host cell response. Which one
of the following interleukins is not derived from T cells?

A   IL-1

B   IL-2

C   IL-3

D   IL-4

E   IL-5

6.28   As humoral immunity plays a huge part in periodontal disease,
which immunoglobulin is found in the greatest quantity in human
serum?

A   IgA

B   IgD

C   IgE

D   IgG

E   IgM

6.27 A

There are two types of IL-1: IL-1α and IL-1β. They are not derived from T cells but from many other cells including macrophages, dendritic cells, some B cells and fibroblasts.

6.28 D

The most prevalent immunoglobulin is IgG, followed by IgA.

6.29 Which teeth are assessed in Ramfjord's index (periodontal disease index)?

A

6		1	4
	4	1	6

B

6			1	4	
	4	1			6

C

	4	1	1	4
	4		1	6

D

6		1		6
6	1	1		6

E

	4	1		6
6			1	4

6.30 When looking at the notes of a patient, you notice that one of the sextants in the BPE has an X. What does this mean?

A A furcation lesion is present

B The dentist was unable to decide what score to give the sextant

C Only two teeth were present in the sextant

D Only one tooth or no teeth were present in the sextant

E Teeth in the sextant are marked for extraction

6.29 B

Ramfjord in 1959 developed an index using data representative of the dentition as a whole. Only having to assess six teeth makes it faster to perform than some other periodontal examinations.

6.30 D

A furcation lesion is indicated by '*'.

A. A furcation lesion is present

6.31 Which one of the following is not a sign of chronic gingivitis?

    A Marginal redness

    B Swelling

    C Bleeding on probing

    D Stippling

    E Increased probing depth

6.32 What is the name for the lesion shown in the figure below?

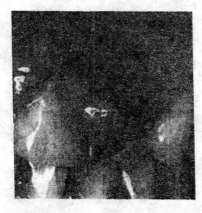

    A Polyp

    B Epulis

    C Abscess

    D Normal anatomy

    E Granuloma

6.31 **D**

In gingivitis there is loss of stippling.

6.32 **B**

The picture shows an epulis.

6.33 Which one of the following is not a potential pathway for initiation or spread of periodontal inflammation?

A Dentinal tubules

B Lateral and accessory root canals

C Cracks and fracture lines

D Iatrogenic perforations

E Poor irrigation during the drilling of restorations

6.34 Which one of the following bacteria involved in periodontal disease is a spirochaete?

A *Porphyromonas gingivalis*

B *Fusobacterium nucleatum*

C *Actinobacillus actinomycetemcomitans*

D *Prevotella intermedia*

E *Treponema denticola*

6.35 Which one of the following is not a local factor in periodontal disease?

A Poor crown margins

B Badly designed partial dentures

C Smoking

D Diabetes

E Mouth breathing

6.33 E

All of the others are putative pathways for periodontal inflammation. Poor irrigation during restorative procedures may lead to pulpal irritation and death, but not periodontal inflammation.

6.34 E

P. gingivalis, *F. nucleatum* and *P. intermedia* are obligate anaerobes. *A. actinomycetemcomitans* is a microaerophilic bacillus. The give away is that the most famous spirochaete, which causes syphilis, is *Treponema pallidum*.

6.35 D

All of the above except pregnancy are local factors, whereas diabetes is a systemic or host factor.

6.36 Which complement component is found in high levels in gingival crevicular fluid and causes chemotaxis and vasodilation?

    A C2

    B C4a

    C C4b

    D C5a

    E C5b

6.37 Which types of micro-organism are found in supragingival plaque?

A	Gram-positive	Gram-negative	Fermentative organisms
B	Aerobic	Gram-negative	Anaerobic bacteria
C	Gram-positive	Aerobic bacteria	Proteolytic bacteria
D	Gram-positive	Aerobic bacteria	Fermentative bacteria
E	Proteolytic bacteria	Gram-negative	Anaerobic bacteria

6.36   D

Cell lysis is only one function (and probably not the most important one) of the complement system. The complement system acts in several ways to mobilise defence mechanisms:

- Opsonization by C3b targets foreign particles for phagocytosis

- Chemotaxis by C5a attracts phagocytic cells to the site of damage. This is aided by the increased permeability of the capillary beds mediated by C3a and C5a. The early complement components are also important for solubilising antigen–antibody complexes, assisting in their catabolism and elimination from the body. Failure of this function can lead to immune complex disorders

- Lysis of antibody-coated cells. (In some cases, this causes more harm than good); complement-mediated lysis can cause serious disorders such as:

  - Rh disease

  - Immune haemolytic anaemia

  - Immune thrombocytopenic purpura

- Promoting antibody formation. Breakdown of C3b generates a fragment (C3d) that binds to antigens enhancing their uptake by dendritic cells and B cells

6.37   D

The most commonly found micro-organisms in supragingival plaque are Gram-positive, aerobic and fermentative bacteria.

6.38 Which types of micro-organism are found in subgingival plaque?

A	Gram-positive	Gram-negative	Fermentative organisms
B	Aerobic	Gram-negative	Anaerobic bacteria
C	Gram-positive	Aerobic bacteria	Proteolytic bacteria
D	Gram-positive	Aerobic bacteria	Fermentative bacteria
E	Proteolytic bacteria	Gram-negative	Anaerobic bacteria

6.39 Which one of the following is not a primary polymorphonuclear leucocyte abnormality that leads to periodontal disease?

A Chediak–Higashi syndrome

B Papillon–Lefèvre syndrome

C Kostmann syndrome

D Haim–Munk syndrome

E Kallmann syndrome

6.38   E

The most commonly found micro-organisms in subgingival plaque are proteolytic, Gram-negative and anaerobic bacteria.

6.39   E

- **Chediak–Higashi syndrome** is a rare autosomal recessive disorder that affects multiple systems of the body, and arises from a mutation in the lysosomal trafficking regulator gene, LYST.

- **Kostmann syndrome**, also known as severe congenital neutropenia (SCN), is a rare inherited form of severe chronic neutropenia, usually detected soon after birth. It was discovered in 1956 by the Swedish doctor Kostmann.

- **Kallmann syndrome** is an example of hypogonadism (decreased functioning of the sex hormone-producing glands) caused by a deficiency of gonadotropin-releasing hormone (GnRH), which is created by the hypothalamus. Kallmann syndrome is also known as hypothalamic hypogonadism, familial hypogonadism with anosmia, or hypogonadotrophic hypogonadism, reflecting its disease mechanism.

6.40 Which one of the following is used to describe a condition in which a human, who is not himself sick, harbours an infective organism which may cause disease in those to whom it is transmitted?

    A Carrier state

    B Homozygous

    C Karyotype

    D Polyzygous

    E Heterozygous

6.41 Which interleukin (IL) is most responsible for neutrophil chemotaxis?

    A IL-1

    B IL-4

    C IL-8

    D IL-15

    E IL-20

6.40 **A**

A carrier is a person who is phenotypically normal but may have an underlying genetic disorder. They may be heterozygotes, they may be homozygotes, but you could not say with any certainty that they are of that genetic state.

6.41 **C**

IL-8 is most responsible for neutrophil chemotaxis.

7.1 Which of the following drugs is likely to cause gingival enlargement?

A Amlodipine

B Bisoprolol

C Candesartan

D Nicorandil

E Propranolol

7.2 Bisphosphonates affect which cell most commonly?

A Cementoblast

B Chondroblast

C Fibroblast

D Osteoblast

E Osteoclast

7.3 Which of the following drugs is associated with altered taste as a side effect?

A Amoxicillin

B Co-amoxiclav

C Chloramphenicol

D Flucloxacillin

E Metronidazole

7.1 A

Common side effects of amlodipine include ankle swelling, dizziness, flushing, headaches, oedema, stomach pain, nausea and tiredness.

7.2 E

Bone undergoes constant turnover and is kept in balance (homeostasis) by osteoblasts creating bone and osteoclasts destroying bone. Bisphosphonates inhibit the digestion of bone by encouraging osteoclasts to undergo apoptosis, or cell death, thereby slowing bone loss.

7.3 E

Oral side effects include candidiasis, altered taste and stomatitis. Other side effects include, dysuria, a disulfiram-like reaction with alcohol and rarely neutropenia.

7.4 The upper limit of the safe dosage of lidocaine without adrenaline in a 50-kg woman is:

    A 100 mg

    B 150 mg

    C 200 mg

    D 250 mg

    E 300 mg

7.5 The speed of onset of a local anaesthetic is most closely associated with which of the following?

    A Lipid binding

    B pK_a

    C Protein binding

    D Volume

    E Weight of patient

7.6 A patient with candidiasis returns to your surgery extremely upset. His INR (international normalised ratio) has altered greatly since you prescribed him a medication. Which of the following medications is likely to cause this issue?

    A Clotrimazole

    B Erythromycin

    C Ketoconazole

    D Miconazole

    E Nystatin

7.4   B

The safe dosage of lidocaine without adrenaline is 3 mg/kg, whereas with adrenaline it is 7 mg/kg.

7.5   C

The pK_a is most closely associated with the speed of onset. If the local anaesthetic has a pH close to 7.4 (tissue pH), then it will start to work faster than a local anaesthetic with a different pH. The potency of the local anaesthetic is associated with increased lipid solubility and duration is associated with protein binding.

7.6   D

Miconazole, similar to warfarin, is hepatically metabolised by cytochrome P450. It interacts with amphotericin B and phenytoin. As structurally it is related to ketoconazole, it may interact with ciclosporin and rifampicin. Miconazole has a high probability of potentiating the hypoprothrombinaemic effects of warfarin by decreasing warfarin's intrinsic clearance and increasing its plasma-free fraction.

7.7 Which one of the following statements regarding paracetamol is true?

A   It is excreted unchanged by the kidney

B   The maximum recommended daily dose in an adult is 4 g

C   It is not antipyretic

D   It inhibits coughing

E   It should not be given in patients allergic to aspirin

7.8 Which one of the following drugs cannot be used in pregnancy?

A   Tetracycline

B   Paracetemol

C   Nystatin

D   Lidocaine

E   Penicillin

7.9 Which one of the following is not a recognised effect of orally administered steroids?

A   Weight loss

B   Osteoporosis

C   Hyperglycaemia

D   Mental disturbances

E   Immunosuppression

7.7   B

Paracetamol is metabolised in the liver, is antipyretic, and does not inhibit coughing.

7.8   A

Tetracycline affects tooth and bone formation. Particularly relevant to dentistry is the brown lines which appear on teeth that were developing during the period of administration of tetracycline.

7.9   A

Steroids cause Cushingoid effects leading to weight gain, osteoporosis, diabetes and immunosuppression.

7.10 Which one of the following statements is **not** true?

A Carbamazepine leads to abnormal liver function tests

B Flumazenil is a benzodiazepine antagonist

C Benzodiazepines are commonly used anxiolytics

D Benzodiazepines are used in the treatment of epilepsy

E Carbamazepine is a benzodiazepine

7.11 Which one of the following statements is correct about local anaesthetics?

A The most commonly used local anaesthetic in dental surgeries is 0.2% lidocaine with 1:80 000 adrenaline

B Lidocaine must be stored below 5 °C

C Lidocaine has a longer lasting effect than bupivacaine

D Lidocaine without adrenaline has a longer lasting effect than lidocaine with adrenaline

E 3% prilocaine with 0.03 IU/ml felypressin is a commonly used dental anaesthetic

7.12 Which one of the following statements is correct about lidocaine?

A A 2.2 ml cartridge of 2% lidocaine contains 4.4 mg of lidocaine

B Lidocaine and prilocaine are esters

C Esters are more likely to cause an allergic reaction than amides

D Amide local anaesthetics are metabolised by the liver

E Prilocaine is more toxic than lidocaine

7.10   E

Carbamazepine is a drug used for trigeminal neuralgia and epilepsy, however it is not a benzodiazepine. It has side effects which include abnormal liver function tests and bone marrow suppression. Benzodiazepines act on the central nervous system and can have hypnotic, anxiolytic, anticonvulsant and sedative effects. Flumazenil is the reversal agent for midazolam and is therefore a benzodiazepine antagonist.

7.11   E

Prilocaine is more commonly known by its trade name Citanest. Lidocaine is normally used as a 2% solution and adrenaline causes the vasoconstriction, leading to increased anaesthesia.

7.12   C

The 2.2 ml cartridge contains 44 mg of lidocaine. Both lidocaine and prilocaine are amides and therefore are less likely to cause an allergic reaction. Lidocaine is a much more toxic drug than prilocaine.

7.13   Which one of the following is not an anti-fungal drug?

    A   Miconazole

    B   Fluconazole

    C   Aciclovir

    D   Nystatin

    E   Itraconazole

7.14   Regarding penicillin, which one of the following statements is incorrect?

    A   Penicillin is the antibiotic of choice for anaerobic infections

    B   It works by interfering with bacterial cell wall synthesis

    C   It is bactericidal

    D   It is antagonistic to tetracycline

    E   It frequently causes allergic reactions

7.15   Which one of the following drugs can be prescribed safely in pregnancy?

    A   Metronidazole

    B   Paracetamol

    C   Prilocaine

    D   Miconazole

    E   Methotrexate

7.13   C

Aciclovir is an anti-viral drug, commonly used topically for herpes simplex. It can also be used more effectively systemically.

7.14   A

Penicillins are a bactericidal group of antibiotics. Their mode of action is to inhibit the cross linking of mucopeptides in cell walls and therefore prevent cell wall synthesis. The drug of choice for anaerobic infections is metronidazole.

7.15   B

Methotrexate can be used to produce an abortion in the early stages of pregnancy. Prilocaine can induce labour, especially when combined with felypressin.

7.16 Which one of the following drugs does not induce gingival hyperplasia?

- **A** Nifedipine
- **B** Carbamazepine
- **C** Phenytoin
- **D** Diltiazem
- **E** Ciclosporin

7.17 Patients who take warfarin should always:

- **A** Carry a purple warning card
- **B** Have a therapeutic range of international normalised ratio (INR) between 2 and 3
- **C** Stop all anti-coagulants 3 days prior to tooth extractions
- **D** Have their blood regularly monitored to measure their INR
- **E** Wear a MedicAlert bracelet

7.18 Which of the following statements regarding tetracyclines is true?

- **A** They are narrow spectrum antibiotics
- **B** They are absorbed better when taken with milk
- **C** They may be used as a mouthwash in a dose of 45 mg dissolved in a little water and held in the mouth
- **D** They cause intrinsic staining of teeth
- **E** They cause extrinsic staining of teeth

7.16   B

Nifedipine and diltiazem are calcium channel blockers, phenytoin is an anti-epileptic and ciclosporin is an immunosuppressant. These all induce gingival hyperplasia.

7.17   D

The warning card is a yellow card, and they do not need to wear a MedicAlert bracelet. Their doctor decides the appropriate level of INR, which may be as much as 4.5 for patients who have had a valve replacement. They may not need to stop their anticoagulants for simple extractions if their INR is below 3.5 as we should be able to cope with this level of haemorrhage.

7.18   D

Tetracyclines should not be given in pregnancy nor in patients who are under 12 years of age. A 250 mg tetracycline capsule can be used as a mouthwash to prevent or treat infected oral ulceration.

7.19 Which one of the following is a sign or a symptom of lidocaine overdose?

  A   Light headedness

  B   Tachycardia

  C   Rash

  D   Hypertension

  E   Hyperventilation

7.20 Which one of the following does not always need to be included on a prescription?

  A   The prescriber's signature

  B   The date of the prescription

  C   The dose of the drug in words

  D   The name and address of the prescriber

  E   The address of the patient

7.21 Lidocaine works by blocking which one of the following channels?

  A   Calcium channels

  B   Sodium channels

  C   Potassium channels

  D   Hydrogen channels

  E   Chloride channels

7.19   A

Signs and symptoms of lidocaine overdose are: respiratory depression, hypotension, bradycardia, confusion, convulsions and light headedness.

7.20   C

Only if the drug being prescribed is a controlled drug does the dose of the drug have to be written in words.

7.21   B

Lidocaine works by blocking sodium channels, and prevents depolarisation of the nerve membranes as it stabilises the membranes.

7.22 Which one of the following statements regarding aspirin is false?

  A   It is a non-steroidal anti-inflammatory drug (NSAID)

  B   It prevents the synthesis of prostaglandin E_2

  C   It has anti-pyretic properties

  D   It is a commonly used analgesic for children

  E   It may cause gastric mucosal irritation and bleeding

7.23 Which one of the following interacts with warfarin to lower the patient's INR?

  A   Fluconazole

  B   Vitamin K

  C   Metronidazole

  D   Erythromycin

  E   Aspirin

7.24 Which one of the following drugs and doses for the treatment of atypical facial pain is not correct?

  A   Dothiepin 75 mg nocte

  B   Amitriptyline 25 mg daily

  C   Fluoxetine 20 mg daily

  D   Flumazenil 20 mg daily

  E   Nortriptyline 25 mg daily

7.22 D

Aspirin is an NSAID which prevents the synthesis of prostaglandin E_2. It has anti-pyretic properties because of its action on the hypothalamus and should be avoided in children due to the possibility of Reye's syndrome.

7.23 B

Fluconazole, metronidazole and erythromycin potentiate warfarin's action. Vitamin K interacts with warfarin but causes a lowering of the INR. Aspirin does not affect the INR as it does not interfere with the clotting cascade, only the function of the platelets.

7.24 D

All of the above except D are used for the treatment of atypical facial pain. Flumazenil is a reversal agent for midazolam and therefore is not used for the treatment of atypical facial pain.

7.25 Which one of the following is not an NSAID?

   A Aspirin

   B Ibuprofen

   C Indometacin

   D Naproxen

   E Paracetamol

7.26 Which one of the following is the mechanism by which erythromycin works?

   A It blocks protein synthesis at the 30S ribosomal subunit

   B It blocks protein synthesis at the 50S ribosomal subunit

   C It blocks mRNA synthesis

   D It blocks peptidoglycan synthesis

   E It blocks cell wall synthesis

7.27 Which one of the following antibiotics can cause pseudomembranous colitis?

   A Amoxicillin

   B Erythromycin

   C Clindamycin

   D Metronidazole

   E Chloramphenicol

7.25   E

All of the above except paracetamol are NSAIDs. Indometacin and naproxen are especially used in rheumatoid arthritis.

7.26   B

Gentamicin works at the 30S subunit, rifampicin blocks mRNA synthesis, vancomycin classically blocks peptidoglycan synthesis and penicillin blocks cell wall synthesis.

7.27   C

Clindamycin causes the death of many commensal organisms in the colon and leads to overgrowth of less favourable organisms causing pseudomembranous colitis, which has a high mortality.

7.28 Which one of the following clotting factors is not affected by warfarin?

    A II

    B VII

    C VIII

    D IX

    E X

7.29 Which one of the following commonly prescribed antibiotics produces a disulfiram-like reaction on ingestion of alcohol?

    A Amoxicillin

    B Erythromycin

    C Clindamycin

    D Metronidazole

    E Chloramphenicol

7.30 Which of the following drug–side effect combinations is correct?

	Drug	Side effect
A	Vancomycin	Red man syndrome
B	Amoxicillin	Pseudomembranous colitis
C	Propranolol	Gingival hyperplasia
D	Paracetamol	Reye's syndrome
E	Erythromycin	Tooth staining

7.28 C

Warfarin affects the extrinsic clotting pathway and prolongs the prothrombin time. It increases bleeding and is teratogenic.

7.29 D

Metronidazole has the classic disulfiram-like reaction with alcohol. Patients should be always advised to avoid alcohol when taking this drug.

7.30 A

Clindamycin causes pseudomembranous colitis; nifedipine or diltiazem are the anti-hypertensives which cause gingival hyperplasia; aspirin, not paracetamol causes Reye's syndrome; and tetracyclines cause tooth staining.

7.31 Which is the most important drug to be administered in an addisonian crisis?

A   Adrenaline

B   Hydrocortisone sodium succinate

C   Prednisolone

D   Chlorphenamine

E   Flumazenil

7.32 Which one of the following is not a side effect of an excess of opioid treatment?

A   Respiratory depression

B   Constipation

C   Addiction

D   Hallucination

E   Dilated pupils

7.33 Which one of the following drugs should not be given to asthmatic people?

A   Metronidazole

B   Amoxicillin

C   Ibuprofen

D   Captopril

E   Paracetamol

7.31   B

A patient having an addisonian crisis has a lack of corticosteroids in their circulation, which leads to collapse. Intravenous hydrocortisone sodium succinate is the drug of choice and will help rectify the situation. Prednisolone is a steroid also, however it is given orally and takes longer to act. Therefore it is ineffectual in an emergency situation.

7.32   E

Miosis or pinpoint pupils is one of the signs of opiate misuse or overdose. All of the other options are correct.

7.33   C

Ibuprofen is contraindicated in asthma as it can cause bronchoconstriction and can precipitate an asthma attack.

7.34 **Which one of the following statements regarding paracetamol is incorrect?**

    A   It is an anti-pyretic

    B   An overdose is treated by *N*-acetylcysteine

    C   It is locally acting

    D   It is hepatotoxic in overdose

    E   It is prescribed in doses of between 500 mg and 1 g four times daily

7.35 **Which one of the following doses of adrenaline in the treatment of anaphylaxis is correct?**

    A   Adrenaline 0.5 ml of 1:100 intramuscularly

    B   Adrenaline 5 ml of 1:100 intramuscularly

    C   Adrenaline 0.5 ml of 1:1000 intramuscularly

    D   Adrenaline 5 ml of 1:1000 intramuscularly

    E   Adrenaline 0.5 ml of 1:10 000 intramuscularly

7.36 **Which one of the following causes a dry mouth?**

    A   Adrenaline

    B   Atropine

    C   Amoxicillin

    D   Anti-malarials

    E   Angiotensin-converting enzyme (ACE) inhibitors

7.34   C

Paracetamol has a systemic action, acts centrally and has an anti-pyretic action. An overdose is hepatotoxic and is treated by *N*-acetylcysteine.

7.35   C

The correct dose is 0.5–1 ml of 1:1000 intramuscularly, with hydrocortisone sodium succinate 200 mg, chlorphenamine 10–30 mg intramuscularly, oxygen and 1–2 litres of colloid.

7.36   B

Atropine is an antimuscarinic drug which leads to the decreased salivary outflow and the dry mouth.

7.37 The most effective drug in the treatment of Parkinson's disease is:

A   Levodopa

B   Sulfasalazine

C   Metoclopramide

D   Bactroban

E   Clopidogrel

7.38 Penicillin is an effective agent against rapidly growing cells because it:

A   Interferes with folinic acid production

B   Inhibits RNA synthesis

C   Inhibits DNA synthesis

D   Inhibits cell wall synthesis

E   Interferes with folate synthesis

7.37 A

Parkinson's disease belongs to a group of conditions called movement disorders. It is characterised by muscle rigidity, tremor, a slowing of physical movement (bradykinesia) and, in extreme cases, a loss of physical movement (akinesia). The primary symptoms are the result of decreased stimulation of the motor cortex by the basal ganglia, usually caused by the insufficient formation and action of dopamine, which is produced in the dopaminergic neurones of the brain. Secondary symptoms may include high-level cognitive dysfunction and subtle language problems. Parkinson's disease is both chronic and progressive and is the most common cause of chronic progressive parkinsonism, a term which refers to the syndrome of tremor, rigidity, bradykinesia and postural instability. Parkinson's disease is also called 'primary parkinsonism' or 'idiopathic Parkinson's disease' (classically meaning having no known cause although many genetic mutations associated with Parkinson's disease have since been discovered). Although many forms of parkinsonism are idiopathic, secondary instances may result from toxicity most notably of drugs, head trauma, or other medical disorders.

7.38 D

β-Lactam antibiotics work by inhibiting the formation of peptidoglycan cross-links in the bacterial cell wall. The β-lactam moiety (functional group) of penicillin binds to the enzyme DD-transpeptidase, which links the peptidoglycan molecules in bacteria, and thus weakens the cell wall of the bacterium (in other words, the antibiotic causes cytolysis or death due to osmotic pressure). In addition, the build-up of peptidoglycan precursors triggers the activation of bacterial cell wall hydrolases and autolysins, which further digest the bacterium's existing peptidoglycan. Gram-positive bacteria are called protoplasts when they lose their cell wall. Gram-negative bacteria do not lose their cell wall completely and are called spheroplasts after treatment with penicillin. Penicillin shows a synergistic effect with aminoglycosides, since the inhibition of peptidoglycan synthesis allows aminoglycosides to penetrate the bacterial cell wall more easily, allowing disruption of bacterial protein synthesis within the cell.

7.39 Sulphonamides are synergistic bacteriostatic agents because in bacteria they:

 A   Interfere with folinic acid production

 B   Inhibit RNA synthesis

 C   Inhibit DNA synthesis

 D   Inhibit cell wall synthesis

 E   Interfere with folate synthesis

7.40 Procaine is an:

 A   Amide

 B   Ester

 C   Benzoate

 D   Hypnotic anxiolytic

 E   Alkylating agent

7.41 Metronidazole:

 A   Interferes with folinic acid production

 B   Inhibits RNA synthesis

 C   Inhibits nucleic acid synthesis

 D   Inhibits cell wall synthesis

 E   Interferes with folate synthesis

7.39   A

In bacteria, antibacterial sulphonamides act as competitive inhibitors of the enzyme dihydropteroate synthetase (DHPS).

7.40   B

Procaine is a local anaesthetic drug of the amino ester group. Procaine is used less frequently today since more effective (and hypoallergenic) alternatives such as lidocaine (Xylocaine) are available. Prior to the discovery of procaine, cocaine was the most commonly used local anaesthetic. Procaine (like cocaine) has the advantage of constricting blood vessels, which reduces bleeding, unlike other local anaesthetics such as lidocaine, but without the euphoric and addictive qualities of cocaine. Procaine is metabolised in the plasma by the enzyme pseudocholinesterase through hydrolysis into para-amino benzoic acid (PABA), which is then excreted by the kidneys into the urine. Allergic reactions to procaine are usually not in response to procaine itself, but to PABA.

7.41   C

Metronidazole is a prodrug. It is converted in anaerobic organisms by the redox enzyme pyruvate-ferredoxin oxidoreductase. The nitro group of metronidazole is chemically reduced by ferredoxin (or a ferredoxin-linked metabolic process) and the products are responsible for disrupting the DNA helical structure, thus inhibiting nucleic acid synthesis. Metronidazole is selectively taken up by anaerobic bacteria and sensitive protozoal organisms because of the ability of these organisms to reduce metronidazole to its active form intracellularly.

7.42 Which topically applied antibiotic can be applied to facial wounds to prevent infection and reduce scarring?

A Penicillin

B Erythromycin

C Chloramphenicol

D Metronidazole

E Fluconazole

7.42   C

Chloramphenicol is frequently applied to facial wounds to reduce infection and prevent scarring.

8
Radiology

8.1 What is the risk of developing a fatal radiation-induced malignancy after having had a bitewing radiograph taken?

A   1 in 2000

B   1 in 200 000

C   1 in 2000 000

D   1 in 20 000 000

E   1 in 200 000 000

8.2 Which of the following has the greatest impact on reducing the amount of radiation to which a patient will be exposed during the taking of a periapical radiograph?

A   The size of the film

B   The use of a film holder

C   The use of circular collimation

D   The use of rectangular collimation

E   The use of a lead apron

8.3 Under the Ionising Radiation (medical exposure) Regulations (IR[ME]R) 2000, which one of the following best describes the three roles that a qualified dental practitioner is automatically entitled to take on?

A   Medical physics expert, operator, referrer

B   Medical physics expert, practitioner, radiation protection adviser

C   Radiation protection adviser, referrer, practitioner

D   Radiation protection adviser, practitioner, operator

E   Referrer, practitioner, operator

8.1 D

The Australian Dental Association estimates this to be the risk of a fatal malignancy.

8.2 D

The use of rectangular collimation has a risk reduction of 61% with regard to a patient developing a fatal malignancy as a result of having had a periapical radiograph. Circular collimation is outdated technology and should not be used. The use of a film holder will reduce patient risk; however, the reduction is not as large as 61%.

8.3 E

The Regulations define the duty holders who carry responsibility under the new Regulations:

- The **employer**, normally the local hospital board/trust in the NHS environment
- The **referrer**, a registered health-care professional who is entitled in accordance with the employer's procedures to refer patients for medical exposures
- The **practitioner**, a registered health-care professional who is entitled in accordance with the employer's procedures and whose primary responsibility is justification of the individual medical exposure
- The **operator**, a person who is entitled in accordance with the employer's procedures to undertake the practical aspects of the medical exposure.
- The **employer**, who has responsibility for creating a framework for radiation protection of the patient through the provision of written standard operating procedures, with which duty holders must comply.

8.4 Which one of the following statements is the correct diagnosis for the condition shown in the X-ray?

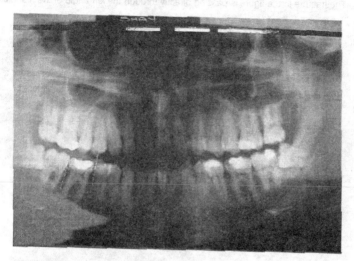

- A Fractured left body of mandible
- B Fractured right body of mandible
- C Fractured left angle of mandible
- D Fractured right angle of mandible
- E Fractured right ramus of mandible

8.5 Which one other X-ray should be taken for the case in Question 8.4?

- A Occipito-mental (OM) 0°
- B OM 30°
- C OM 50°
- D Postero-anterior (PA) mandible
- E Antero-posterior (AP) mandible

8.4 C

The fracture in the figure is passing directly through the left angle of the mandible.

8.5 D

With every fracture two views should be taken, and the appropriate X-rays for a fractured mandible are an orthopantomogram (OPG) and a PA mandible.

8.6 If the patient had a 'bucket handle' fracture, what would the fracture be?

A   A unilateral condylar fracture

B   A bilateral condylar fracture

C   A unilateral body of mandible fracture

D   A bilateral parasymphysial fracture

E   A fracture of the angle of the mandible and a contralateral condylar fracture

8.7 Post-operatively, the patient in Question 8.4 has anaesthesia of a very small circular area on the chin. However, they have full sensation of the lip. Which one of the statements below correctly explains this deficit in sensation?

A   The lingual nerve has cross-over with the inferior dental nerve leading to an anomaly in sensation

B   The nerve to stylohyoid has been damaged

C   The marginal mandibular branch of the facial nerve has been damaged

D   The mental nerve has been damaged

E   A few aberrant nerve fibres from the nerve to mylohyoid have been stretched during retraction leading to anaesthesia of the chin

8.6   D

This is known as a bucket handle fracture because the unfavourable muscle pull causes the anterior fragment to be pulled downwards leading to the appearance of a bucket handle. If a patient has a fracture of the body, angle or ramus of the mandible, it is always worth paying attention to the contralateral side as there may well be a condylar fracture, especially if the cause of the injury is inter-personal violence.

8.7   E

Occasionally some aberrant nerve fibres from the nerve to mylohyoid are present in the mental region, leading to a paraesthesia or anaesthesia of a small area on the chin when retraction occurs during ORIF (open reduction internal fixation). If the mental nerve had been damaged there would be a loss of sensation to the lip. If the marginal mandibular branch of the facial nerve had been damaged there would be drooping of the corner of the mouth, but no loss of sensation.

8.8   Which one of the following statements is the correct diagnosis for
       the condition shown in the X-ray?

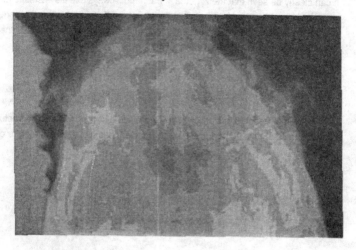

    A   Fractured mandible
    B   Fractured nasal bones
    C   Fractured maxilla
    D   Fractured zygoma
    E   Le Fort II fracture

8.9   What other X-rays should be taken for the patient in Question 8.8?
    A   OM 0°
    B   OM 50°
    C   Reverse Towne's
    D   PA mandible
    E   AP mandible

8.8   D

It can clearly be seen that the zygoma is fractured. Always use a systematic method when looking at X-rays. Always start at the top of the X-ray, and follow the bones to see if there are any discrepancies or discontinuities and compare with the other side. This is a very easy way of interpreting X-rays.

8.9   A

The X-ray in Question 8.8 is an OM 30°. To provide a second view of the fracture, an OM 0° should always be performed when a patient has a suspected fracture of the zygoma.

8.10 When a patient has a fractured zygoma, which nerve is commonly damaged, leading to a paraesthesia or anaesthesia?

A Inferior dental nerve

B Facial nerve

C Infraorbital nerve

D Supraorbital nerve

E Supratrochlear nerve

8.11 Which eponymous hook is commonly used to reduce the fracture in the patient in Question 8.10?

A Barnes

B Gillies

C Howarth

D Bowdler–Henry

E McIndoe

8.12 Which one of the following is not a complication of a fractured zygoma?

A Diplopia

B Infraorbital nerve paraesthesia

C Trismus

D Subconjunctival haemorrhage

E Facial nerve palsy

8.10 C

The infraorbital nerve is commonly damaged, leading to paraesthesia or anaesthesia. Rarely there is permanent damage to the nerve structure, and the vast majority of patients recover.

8.11 B

The Gillies hook is commonly used to reduce the fractured zygoma into its correct anatomical position. Howarth, Bowdler–Henry and McIndoe are also eponymous instruments.

8.12 E

Facial nerve palsy is usually produced by wounding with a sharp weapon such as a knife or a broken glass. Trismus occurs with fractured zygomas because the masseter is attached to the zygomatic arch.

8.13 What is unusual about this X-ray?

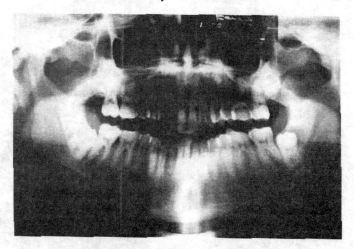

   A There is a dentigerous cyst present

   B There is a supernumerary present in the maxillary arch

   C There is a supernumerary present in the mandibular arch

   D There is a three rooted mandibular first molar

   E There is nothing unusual

8.14 Which one of the following things would you not warn the patient about when consenting for extraction of the supernumerary, the mandibular first molar and mandibular third molar?

   A Paraesthesia/anaesthesia of the inferior dental nerve

   B Paraesthesia/anaesthesia of the lingual nerve

   C Paraesthesia/anaesthesia of the facial nerve

   D Pain, swelling and bruising

   E Antibiotics given may interfere with the contraceptive pill

8.13 E

There is nothing unusual about this radiograph.

8.14 C

All other statements are valid complications of the procedure described.

8.15   Which one of the following radiographic features would not suggest
        that the patient would be at high risk of damage to their inferior
        dental (ID) nerve during the removal of a mandibular third molar?

        A   Loss of the tramlines of the ID canal

        B   Deviation of the tramlines of the ID canal

        C   Widening of the tramlines of the ID canal

        D   Narrowing of the tramlines of the ID canal

        E   Radiolucent band across the tooth

8.16   What is the radiation exposure when taking an OPG?

        A   0.001 mSv

        B   0.01 mSv

        C   0.1 mSv

        D   1.0 mSv

        E   10.0 mSv

8.17   Which of the following is the most commonly associated pathology
        with wisdom teeth?

        A   Pericoronitis

        B   Mesioangular impaction

        C   Distoangular impaction

        D   Horizontal impaction

        E   Cystic change

8.15 C

All of the other radiographic features indicate that the patient is at high risk of damage to their ID nerve during extraction of their mandibular third molar.

8.16 B

The radiation exposure when taking an OPG is 0.01 mSv.

8.17 A

Pericoronitis is one of the most common presentations of pain with wisdom teeth. It is inflammation of the operculum, which is soft tissue, therefore does not show radiographically. Mesioangular impaction > distoangular impaction > horizontal impaction.

8.18 Which type of cyst is present on the X-ray below?

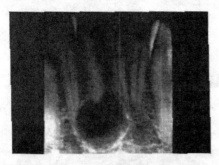

    A   Eruption cyst

    B   Odontogenic keratocyst

    C   Dentigerous cyst

    D   Apical periodontal cyst

    E   Lateral periodontal cyst

8.19 What other X-ray may be appropriate when assessing cysts in the mandible?

    A   PA mandible

    B   AP mandible

    C   OM 0°

    D   Lower occlusal

    E   Reverse Towne's

8.20 If the cyst in Question 8.18 was multilocular, what would be the more likely diagnosis?

    A   Eruption cyst

    B   Odontogenic keratocyst

    C   Dentigerous cyst

    D   Eruption cyst

    E   Lateral periodontal cyst

8.18 D

Apical periodontal cysts are the most common cyst to be found as an incidental finding on an X-ray.

8.19 D

The lower occlusal enables you to assess the bucco-lingual expansion of the cyst.

8.20 B

Odontogenic keratocysts are commonly multilocular and have a high rate of recurrence.

8.21 **Which syndrome is associated with odontogenic keratocysts?**

   A   Gorlin–Goltz

   B   Peutz–Jeghers

   C   Gardner's syndrome

   D   Apert's syndrome

   E   Horner's syndrome

8.22 **Where are odontogenic keratocysts most commonly found?**

   A   Maxillary antrum

   B   Mandibular third molar region

   C   Mandibular anterior region

   D   Maxillary anterior region

   E   None of the above

8.23 **Which of the following statements regarding processing radiographs is true?**

   A   The developer is an acidic solution

   B   The developer needs changing daily

   C   Fixation is the process by which silver halide crystals are removed to reveal the white areas on the film

   D   The lower the temperature of the developer solution, the faster the film will be developed

   E   If the film is not left in the developer long enough then the radiograph will be too dark

8.21 A

Odontogenic keratocysts are associated with Gorlin–Goltz syndrome. This syndrome consists of fronto-temporal bossing, calcified falx cerebri and multiple basal cell naevi.

8.22 B

Odontogenic keratocysts occur most frequently in the mandibular third molar region.

8.23 C

The developer is an alkali solution, which is oxidised by air, and needs changing only every 10 days or so. If the film is not left in the developer long enough it will be too light, as not enough silver will be deposited on it.

8.24 In order to limit the dose for a periapical radiograph:

  A Use a low-speed film

  B Use a lead apron

  C Use the optimal voltage (700 kV)

  D Use the bisecting angle technique

  E Use a rectangular collimator

8.25 The correct order of the stages of processing radiographic film is:

  A Developing, washing, fixing, washing, drying

  B Fixation, washing, developing, washing, drying

  C Washing, developing, washing, fixation, drying

  D Washing, fixing, washing, developing, drying

  E Washing, developing, fixation, washing, drying

8.26 Which one of the following annual dose limits is the correct Ionising Radiation Regulations (IRR) 1999 limit?

  A General public – 2 mSv

  B Non-classified workers – 2 mSv

  C Non-classified workers – 20 mSv

  D Classified workers – 2 mSv

  E Classified workers – 20 mSv

8.24 E

The use of a rectangular collimator decreases the dose of radiation by 50%. Lead aprons are not used anymore and are no longer recommended. The optimal voltage is 70 kV and a fast-speed film should be used.

8.25 A

Remember that the film needs to washed between developing and fixation, and the fixative needs to be washed off before drying.

8.26 E

The IRR 1999 annual dose limits are:

- Classified workers – 20 mSv
- Non-classified workers – 6 mSv
- General public – 1 mSv

8.27 Which one of the following lesions would not present as a multi-locular radiolucent lesion in the mandible?

    A   Ameloblastoma

    B   Calcifying epithelial odontogenic tumour (CEOT)

    C   Odontogenic keratocyst

    D   Odontogenic myxoma

    E   Aneurysmal bone cyst

8.28 Which one of the following lesions would not present as a radiopaque lesion in the mandible?

    A   CEOT

    B   Submandibular salivary calculus

    C   Cemento-osseous dysplasia

    D   Complex odontoma

    E   Odontogenic fibroma

8.29 Which one of the following lesions could present as a unilocular radiolucent lesion in the mandible?

    A   Dentigerous cyst

    B   Ameloblastoma

    C   Stafne's bone cavity

    D   Ameloblastic fibroma

    E   All of the above

8.27   B

A CEOT is a radiopaque lesion, owing to its calcifying nature.

8.28   E

All of the other lesions are radiopaque.

8.29   E

All of the above lesions can present as a unilocular radiolucent lesion in the mandible.

8.30 **What type of filter is used in X-ray machines?**

    A Tungsten

    B Tin

    C Copper

    D Molybdenum

    E Aluminium

8.31 **Which part of the X-ray machine performs the following function: 'It removes the peripheral X-rays, therefore minimising the dose to the patient'?**

    A Collimator

    B Filter

    C Imagine intensifier

    D Generator

    E Ion chamber

8.32 **What is the optimal shape for a collimator?**

    A Round

    B Rectangular

    C Square

    D Hexagonal

    E Circular

8.30   E

Aluminium is the material which is most frequently used as the filter in X-ray machines. It is the most efficacious of materials for this purpose.

8.31   A

Collimators are found in linear accelerators used for radiotherapy. They help to shape the beam of radiation emerging from the machine, and they can limit the maximum field size of a beam. The treatment head of a linear accelerator consists of both a primary and secondary collimator. The primary collimator is positioned after the electron beam has reached vertical orientation. When using photons, the primary collimator is placed after the beam has passed through the X-ray target. The secondary collimator is positioned after either a flattening filter (for photon therapy) or a scattering foil (for electron therapy). The secondary collimator consists of two jaws which can be moved to either enlarge or reduce the size of the treatment field. New systems involving multileaf collimators (MLCs) are used to further shape a beam to localise treatment fields in radiotherapy. MLCs consist of approximately 50–120 leaves of heavy, metal collimator plates which slide into place to form the desired field shape.

8.32   C

A square is the most optimal shape for a collimator. A collimator is a device that narrows a beam of particles or waves. To 'narrow' can mean either to cause the directions of motion to become more aligned in a specific direction (i.e. collimated or parallel) or to cause the spatial cross-section of the beam to become smaller.

8.33 What is the radiation dose to a patient in milli-Sieverts (mSv) associated with having an orthopantomogram (OPG)?

    A   0.034

    B   0.34

    C   3.4

    D   34

    E   340

8.34 Which one of the following does NOT support the ALARA principle?

    A   Minimising errors

    B   Slow-speed film

    C   Aluminium filter

    D   Timer

    E   Collimator

8.35 What injury is depicted in the image below?

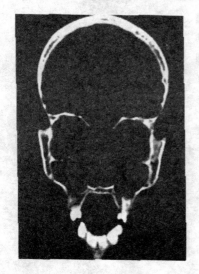

    A   Left orbit fracture

    B   Right orbit fracture

    C   Left zygomatic arch fracture

    D   Right zygomatic arch fracture

    E   Right mandibular fracture

8.33   A

The natural yearly background radiation dosage on average is 1–3 mSv. An OPG provides the same amount of background radiation as a transatlantic flight.

8.34   B

ALARA stands for: As Low as Reasonably Achievable (social and economic factors being taken into account). This term was introduced by the International Commission on Radiological Protection and requires that all be reasonably done to lower radiation exposures below dose limits. Use of fast-speed films means that exposure times can be reduced.

8.35   A

The image shows a left orbital floor fracture. It is very important to correctly 'side' the injury.

9
Restorative Dentistry

9.1 A 32-year-old woman presents with a fractured, vital, maxillary, second premolar with only the palatal cusp remaining. Which one of the following would be the most appropriate restoration?

A Composite restoration

B Porcelain-bonded crown

C Porcelain inlay

D Porcelain onlay

E Porcelain jacket crown

9.2 An 80-year-old patient is complaining that her 20-year-old complete dentures are very worn. On examination you note that the polished surfaces are satisfactory and the freeway space is 4 mm. Which one of the following would be the most appropriate treatment option?

A Copy dentures

B Implant retained maxillary and mandibular dentures

C Implant retained mandibular denture and conventional maxillary denture

D New conventional complete/complete dentures

E Reline of existing dentures

9.3 A patient is referred to the oral surgery department with an apical area on a maxillary central incisor that has a post crown, but no root canal treatment. What is the appropriate course of treatment?

A Oral antibiotics

B Extraction under local anaesthetic

C Retrograde root canal treatment with amalgam

D Retrograde root canal treatment with MTA (mineral trioxide aggregate)

E Orthograde root canal treatment

9.4 Which one of the following cannot be changed during construction of a set of complete dentures?

A Condylar guidance angle

B Curve of Spee

C Cuspal angle

D Freeway space

E Path of insertion

9.1 D

A porcelain onlay is the most appropriate treatment because it is (1) the least destructive method and (2) indirectly manufactured and gives the best aesthetic and functional outcome.

9.2 A

It is unlikely to be possible to place implants in an 80-year-old patient, due to the bone levels and normally his or her general health. The reline of the existing dentures would be appropriate if the patient was complaining of mobility. Copy dentures have the highest success rate in this situation.

9.3 E

Orthograde root canal treatment of a non-root-treated central incisor has the best rate of outcome for the tooth; however, it may not be the cheapest option.

9.4 A

Condylar guidance angle is defined as 'the angle at which the condyle moves away from a horizontal reference plane'. Therefore the condyle cannot be altered when making new dentures. All of the other options can be altered during denture construction.

9.5 What is the file used to explore the apical third of a canal called?

A Searcher

B Seeker

C Finder

D Endodontic explorer

E Endodontic probe

9.6 The file used to explore the apical third of a tooth is usually:

A Size 3-5

B Size 8-10

C Size 15-20

D Size 25-30

E Size 40-50

9.7 Which one of the following are you not looking for when you are exploring the apical third of a canal?

A Hypercementosis

B Branches

C Lateral canals

D Internal root resorption

E Obstruction

9.5 B

The file used to explore the apical third of a canal is called a seeker.

9.6 B

The size 8–10 file is appropriate for the apex of a tooth.

9.7 A

Hypercementosis is found on the root surface of a tooth rather than inside the root canal. All of the others can be found within the canal.

9.8 The root canal you are working on is curved, and you have pre-curved the file accordingly. How can you best tell the direction the file is pointing within the root?

A By mentally noting which direction the file is curved when inserting it

B By looking at the position of the number on the side of the file

C By cutting a notch on the rubber stop

D By taking an intraoral periapical (IOPA) radiograph

E By tactile sensation

9.9 If a canal is narrow, which one of the following can be used to make exploration easier?

A Water

B Bleach

C EDTA

D Calcium hydroxide

E Ferric sulphate

9.10 In a straight-canal tooth, how much should the apical 1 mm be prepared to?

A The size of the first file which binds in that region

B Two to three sizes larger than the first file which binds within that region

C A size 30 file

D A size 40 file

E Depends on the tooth

9.8   C

By cutting a notch in the rubber stop, you can tell which way the canal is curved. An IOPA is unnecessary for this purpose as it only gives you a two-dimensional view of a three-dimensional object.

9.9   C

EDTA is a chelating agent which helps open partially sclerosed or narrow canals. Bleach would not help in exploration of the canal, but it would aid in the destruction of bacteria within the canals.

9.10   B

Ideally the apical 1 mm should be prepared to two to three file sizes larger than the first file which binds in that area. This is because the infected dentine in that region needs to be removed enough to clean the area, but without compromising the apical seal.

9.11 In the apical third of a tooth what percentage of canals are curved?

    A   5%

    B   30%

    C   60%

    D   90%

    E   100%

9.12 What technique is usually used for the production of an apical flare with hand files?

    A   Crown down

    B   Step down

    C   Tug back

    D   Step back

    E   Step up

9.13 To create an apical flare, larger files are used at decreasing lengths. How much difference should there be between the lengths?

    A   0.5 mm

    B   1 mm

    C   1.5 mm

    D   2 mm

    E   3 mm

9.11   D

90% of teeth have some form of curve in the apical third.

9.12   D

Step back is the most recognised method of producing an apical flare with hand instruments. Crown down is the accepted method of producing apical flare with rotary instruments. Tug back is the accepted method to find the apex of a tooth using tactile sensation.

9.13   B

This is optimal to produce a good apical flare.

9.14 **What is the master apical file?**

A A file used to measure the length of the root

B A file used to clear debris from the apical region

C The first file which binds at the working length

D The file used to set the final diameter of the apical region preparation

E The file used to remove pulp material from the canal

9.15 **What is patency filing?**

A A small file is pushed through the apex to keep it clear of debris

B A small file is used circumferentially on canal walls to prevent lateral canals getting blocked

C A nickel titanium rotary file is used to remove debris from the canal, keeping it clear

D A small file is used with bleach to clean the canal

E A small file is used to open the coronal part of the canal

9.16 **Which of the following features is the most important in giving a canal resistance form?**

A Apical stop

B Apical seat

C Open apex

D Natural anatomy

E Tapering of canal walls

9.14 D

A barbed brooch is used to remove pulpal material from the canal. The file used to measure the length of the root is called working length file.

9.15 A

Patency filing is when a small file is pushed through the apex to clear it of debris.

9.16 E

If you taper the canals, it gives them a good resistance form.

9.17 A canal is prepared apically to a size 50 file. No files between size 30 and 50 can pass beyond the length. What type of apical preparation is this?

A Apical stop

B Apical seat

C Open apex

D Closed apex

E Apical stricture

9.18 Which one of the following would you not use to make an apical flare?

A K-flex

B Ni-Ti rotary

C GT (Greater Taper)

D X-files

E Hand files

9.19 Which one of the following is not relevant with regard to using rubber dam?

A Latex allergy

B Sleep apnoea

C Claustrophobia

D Sinusitis

E Emphysema

9.17 A

This describes the preparation of an apical stop.

9.18 D

All the others are genuine endodontic files – the X-files are not.

9.19 B

As rubber dam is made of latex, A is very important. Also, patients can feel claustrophobic when rubber dam is used. If a patient has sinusitis, they will have difficulty breathing through their nose, and having their mouths covered will be problematic. Patients with emphysema should not have anything impairing their airway, as they struggle for oxygen intake at the best of times.

9.20 **Which one of the following is not a function of rubber dam with regard to endodontics?**

A Decreases salivary contamination

B Increases visibility

C Contains excess irrigants

D Makes pulpal access easier

E Decreases medico-legal liability

9.21 **If you cannot manage to place a rubber dam on a tooth, which one of the following solutions is unacceptable?**

A Parachute chain

B Crown lengthening

C No dam

D Restore using a copper band

E Placing the clamp beaks directly onto the gingivae

9.22 **Which one of the following is not a form of calcium hydroxide?**

A Life

B Dycal

C Hypocal

D Coltosol

E Apexit

9.20   D

Although rubber dam increases visibility, it can sometimes make drilling the access cavity more difficult.

9.21   C

Parachute chain can be used to secure endodontic instruments to prevent aspiration. Crown lengthening and the use of a copper band can facilitate the placement of the clamp. It is not ideal to place the beaks directly onto the gingivae, although it is done in practice. Placing the beaks on the gingivae can cause trauma which will cause pain to the patient later, and in rare cases may cause permanent damage.

9.22   D

Coltosol is a non-eugenol temporary restorative material. Apexit is an endodontic sealer. Dycal and Life are lining materials which can be used on minimal pulpal exposures. Hypocal is non-setting calcium hydroxide.

9.23 Which one of the following statements about root caries is false?

A   It is more common in patients with reduced salivary flow than those with normal salivary flow

B   It is frequently managed with topical fluoride

C   It is frequently managed with systemic fluoride

D   It may be managed without a restoration

E   It occurs more frequently in males than in females

9.24 Which one of the following statements about tooth surface wear is correct?

A   Attrition is tooth surface wear by non-bacterial chemical dissolution

B   Abrasion is tooth wear by other teeth

C   Attrition is tooth surface wear by surfaces other than teeth

D   Erosion is tooth surface wear by non-bacterial chemical dissolution

E   Erosion is tooth surface wear by surfaces other than teeth

9.25 Which one of the following statements about tooth surface loss is correct?

A   Abrasion is characterised by smooth wear facets

B   Erosion is characterised by smooth wear facets

C   Abrasion is the commonest type of wear in young patients

D   Abfraction is caused by stresses around the cervical margins due to flexure of teeth

E   Erosion by gastric acid is usually seen on the labial aspects of upper teeth

9.23   C

Root caries is found more frequently in men than women, in patients who are elderly and in those who have reduced salivary flow. It can be treated with topical fluoride and restorations or may be monitored if the caries has arrested.

9.24   D

Abrasion is tooth surface wear by surfaces other than teeth. Attrition is tooth surface wear by other teeth.

9.25   D

Attrition is characterised by smooth wear facets. The most common type of tooth wear in the young is erosion due to diet. Erosion by gastric acid is commonly seen on the palatal surfaces of upper anterior teeth, especially in bulimic patients.

9.26 **Which one of the following is not a method of monitoring tooth surface loss?**

A Dietary sheets

B Study models

C Smith and Knight indices

D Laser scanning

E Clinical photographs

9.27 **The desirable degree of taper of a preparation to receive a cast restoration is:**

A Less than 2°

B 2–4°

C 5–7°

D 8–12°

E Greater than 12°

9.28 **Which one of the following statements is true?**

A Enamel contains 92% hydroxyapatite by weight

B Enamel is thinnest where it overlies the cusps

C Diamond burs remove enamel by fracturing it

D Tungsten carbide burs remove enamel by grinding

E Stresses within a cavity preparation can be minimised by rounding the internal angle lines

9.26   A

Dietary sheets are used to find the cause of the tooth surface loss, but do not monitor it.

9.27   C

The closer to parallel the walls of the preparation, the greater the resistance to placement. However, a taper of 5–7° is acceptable.

9.28   E

Enamel is 97% hydroxyapatite by weight. Diamond burs grind away enamel and tungsten carbide burs fracture enamel. Enamel is thickest over the cusps.

9.29 Which one of the following statements regarding surgical endodontics is true?

A It is indicated for all failed root canal treatments

B It is not indicated for patients who have pulp stones

C It is indicated to prevent removal of extensive coronal restorative work

D It is indicated in the presence of a periapical radiolucency

E It is contraindicated in multirooted teeth

9.30 Which one of the following problems occurs because of a reduced vertical dimension?

A Difficulty with 'S' sounds

B Poor appearance, showing far too much teeth

C Clicking of teeth when talking

D Sunken lower face, elderly looking appearance

E Poorly located pain in the lower denture bearing area that is relieved when the denture is removed

9.31 Which one of the following statements regarding overdentures is incorrect?

A They are contraindicated in patients with cleft palates

B They are contraindicated in patients with inadequate interarch space

C They are contraindicated in patients with uncontrolled periodontal disease

D They may be indicated when converting a partially dentate patient into a complete denture wearer

E They may be indicated in patients with attrition

9.29 C

Apicectomy can be performed in teeth with extensive coronal restoration work and pulp stones, and can be performed in multirooted teeth. However, the percentage of success dramatically decreases in these teeth.

9.30 D

Patients with reduced vertical dimension will have a sunken appearance.

9.31 A

The contraindications for overdentures are poor oral hygiene, rampant caries and uncontrolled periodontal disease.

9.32   Which one of the following statements regarding Kennedy's
        classification for partially edentulous arches is correct?

   A   A patient with upper right 876543 and an edentulous upper left region
        would be described as a Kennedy Class IV

   B   A patient with lower right 543 and lower left 543 would be classified as
        Kennedy Class IV

   C   A patient with lower right 76 21 and lower left 123 567 would be classified
        as Kennedy Class II

   D   A patient with lower right 76 21 and lower left 123 567 would be classified
        as Kennedy Class III modification 1

   E   A patient with lower right 87654321 and lower left 123 would be
        described as Kennedy Class III

9.33   Which one of the following statements regarding surveying of casts
        for denture design is correct?

   A   It is carried out for complete and partial dentures

   B   It is carried out for complete dentures

   C   It can determine the occluso-vertical dimension

   D   It can be used to determine undercuts with regard to the path of insertion
        of a denture

   E   It is always carried out with the model at right angles to the analyser rod

9.34   Which one of the following statements regarding partial denture
        clasps is true?

   A   In order to be functional they must be resisted by a non-retentive clasp
        arm

   B   Cast cobalt-chrome clasps need to engage undercuts of greater than
        0.5 mm

   C   Stainless steel clasps are more flexible than gold clasps

   D   The longer the clasp, the less flexible it will be

   E   Gingivally approaching clasps are more conspicuous than occlusally
        approaching clasps

9.32   D

- Kennedy Class I – bilateral free end saddle
- Kennedy Class II – unilateral free end saddle
- Kennedy Class III – unilateral bounded saddle
- Kennedy Class IV – a single bounded saddle anterior to the abutment teeth

A modification or other additional edentulous area can be added to Classes I–III when there are other missing teeth.

9.33   D

Surveying is only carried out for partial dentures, and is used to determine a path of insertion and guide-planes.

9.34   A

Cast cobalt-chrome clasps need to engage undercuts of less than 0.25 mm. Gold is more flexible than stainless steel, and the greater the length of clasp, the greater the flexibility.

9.35 Which one of the following is not an advantage of having an over-denture rather than complete dentures?

A Better aesthetics

B Preservation of alveolar bone

C Better sensory feedback

D Increased biting forces

E More reproducible retruded jaw relations

9.36 The depth of reduction of the marginal ridge for an occlusal rest seat in a removable partial denture construction is:

A 0.5 mm

B 1.5 mm

C 3.0 mm

D 5.0 mm

E None of the above

9.37 Cross-arch stabilisation is the main function of which one of the following parts of a removable partial denture?

A Major connector

B Minor connector

C Bracing arm

D Rest seat

E Indirect retainer

9.35   A

Complete dentures and over-dentures have the same aesthetic appeal. By retaining roots, the alveolar bone is retained and there is increased proprioception. By having greater retention from the abutments, the patient is able to produce increased biting forces compared with the complete denture wearer.

9.36   B

The most optimal rest seat reduction is 1.5 mm. If less reduction is performed, then the rest seat will struggle to retain. If there is greater reduction then the tooth structure may be compromised.

9.37   A

The parts of a removable partial denture (RPD) are described below.

- Major connector is the major part that connects the prosthetic teeth together
- Minor connectors are the small struts protruding from the lingual bar at roughly 90 degree angles
- Direct retainer – the clasp arms act to hug the teeth and keep the RPD in place.
- Indirect retainer – the physical retainer is a mesh of metal that allows the pink base material to connect to the metal framework of the RPD. Some consider physical retainers a component in their own category, whereas others consider them within the indirect retainer category (thus making a total of six components)
- Base is the pink material, mimicking gingiva
- Teeth – plastic or porcelain formed in the shape of teeth

9.38 All clasp assemblies should not have:

A One area of retention

B Two areas of retention

C A guide plane

D A bracing element

E Rest seat

9.38   B

Direct retainers come in various designs.

- Cast circumferential clasp (suprabulge):

    Akers'

    Half and half

    Back-action

    – Ring clasp

- Wrought wire clasp

- Roach clasp (infrabulge):

    – I-bar

    – T-bar

    – Y-bar

    – 7-bar

Both cast circumferential and wrought wire clasps are suprabulge clasps, in that they engage an undercut on the tooth by originating coronal to the height of contour, while Roach clasps are infrabulge clasps and engage undercuts by approaching from the gingival.

9.39 A denture which has bilateral free-ended partially edentulous saddles is classified as:

A Kennedy Class I

B Kennedy Class II

C Kennedy Class III

D Kennedy Class IV

E Kennedy Class V

9.39 A

Depending on where in the mouth the teeth are missing, edentulous situations can be grouped under four different categories, as defined by Dr Edward Kennedy in his classification of partially edentulous arches:

- Class I – bilateral free ended partially edentulous
- Class II – unilateral free ended partially edentulous
- Class III – unilateral bounded partially edentulous
- Class IV – bilateral bounded anterior partially edentulous

Kennedy Class I RPDs are fabricated for people who are missing some or all of their posterior teeth on both sides (left and right) in a single arch (either mandibular or maxillary), and there are no teeth posterior to the edentulous area. In other words, Class I RPDs clasp onto teeth that are more towards the front of the mouth, while replacing the missing more-back-of-the-mouth teeth on both sides with false denture teeth. The denture teeth are composed of either plastic or porcelain. Class II RPDs are fabricated for people who are missing some or all of their posterior teeth on one side (left or right) in a single arch, and there are no teeth behind the edentulous area. Thus, Class II RPDs clasp onto teeth that are more towards the front of the mouth, as well as on teeth that are more towards the back of the mouth of the side on which teeth are not missing, while replacing the missing more-back-of-the-mouth teeth on one side with false denture teeth. Class III RPDs are fabricated for people who are missing some teeth such that the edentulous area has teeth remaining both posterior and anterior to it. Unlike Class I and Class II RPDs, which are both tooth-and-tissue-borne (meaning they both clasp onto teeth, as well as rest on the posterior edentulous area for support), Class III RPDs are strictly tooth-borne, which means they only clasp onto teeth and do not need to rest on the tissue for added support. This makes Class III RPDs much more secure as per the three rules of removable prostheses, namely: support, stability and retention. However, if the edentulous area described above crosses the anterior midline (that is, at least both central incisors are missing), the RPD is classified as a Class IV RPD. By definition, a Kennedy Class IV RPD design will possess only one edentulous area.

9.40 Fill in the gap in the following statement: Any clasp assembly must satisfy the basic principle of clasp design that the tooth must be encircled by that clasp by a minimum of ... degrees of the greater circumference of the crown of the tooth passing from diverging axial surfaces to the converging axial surface.

A   80

B   160

C   180

D   270

E   300

9.41 A rest for a removable partial denture must be designed to:

A   Transmit force horizontally on an abutment

B   Transmit force along the long axis of the tooth

C   Prevent the clasp slipping cervically on a tooth

D   Answer A and Answer C

E   Answer B and Answer C

9.40 C

A clasp must encircle the tooth by a minimum of 180 degrees to provide adequate retention.

9.41 E

Rest seats are designed to transmit the force along the long axis of the tooth and also to prevent the clasp slipping cervically on a tooth.

10
Human Disease

10.1 Which one of the following is the most likely viral agent causing unilateral maxillary pain and a sore ear with vesicles in a 45-year-old man?

A   Coxsackie A virus

B   Cytomegalovirus

C   Epstein–Barr Virus

D   Herpes labialis

E   Herpes zoster

10.2 How does glyceryl trinitrate work?

A   Analgesic action

B   Dilates veins and reduces preload

C   Increases preload to the heart by constricting veins

D   Reduces heart rate

E   Reduces potassium levels

10.3 Which of the following treatments would be the most appropriate for a patient who is undergoing a prolonged epileptic seizure?

A   Clonazepam

B   Diazepam

C   Flumazenil

D   Midazolam

E   Temazepam

10.4 At lunchtime you go out to the reception area and find your receptionist unresponsive and collapsed on the floor. What is your initial action?

A   Call 999

B   Call for help

C   Give two rescue breaths

D   Give 30 chest compressions

E   Use the defibrillator

10.1   E

Herpes zoster can cause a manifestation called Ramsay–Hunt syndrome which leads to vesicles being present on the ear. This can also lead to facial nerve palsy and deafness.

10.2   B

Glyceryl trinitrate is a drug that is applied sublingually. It is rapidly absorbed and causes venous dilatation, which in turn reduces venous return to the heart, and therefore decreases preload. As a result of this the heart has a reduced inotropic effect, which will lead to the reduced angina.

10.3   D

Buccal midazolam is most commonly given 5 min after the start of a tonic–clonic seizure. It is important to time when a seizure starts, so that you know when to give the midazolam. It has been licensed and is more predictable than rectal or intramuscular diazepam. Flumazenil is the reversal agent.

10.4   B

The 2010 Resuscitation Council's adult Basic Life Support (BLS) algorithm is:

- Unresponsive – if so call for help
- Open airway
- If not breathing normally dial 999
- Give 2 rescue breaths followed by 30 chest compressions.

10.5 A 28-year-old individual with type 1 diabetes mellitus is found unconscious in the reception area. Which one of the following would be the most appropriate first-line management in a general dental practice setting?

A   2.5 mg glucagon intravenously

B   1.0 mg glucagon intramuscularly

C   2.5 mg glucagon intramuscularly

D   10 ml glucose intravenously

E   100 ml glucose intravenously

10.6 Which one of the following cranial nerves is most likely to be affected in a patient who has lost her corneal reflex?

A   Accessory

B   Abducent

C   Facial

D   Oculomotor

D   Optic

10.7 Which one of the following best describes the main action of warfarin?

A   Affects platelet function

B   Binds via the von Willebrand factor

C   Prolongs the activated partial thromboplastin time

D   Prolongs the bleeding time

E   Prolongs the prothrombin time

10.5 B

Management of hypoglycaemia:

- 1.0 mg glucagon i.m.; repeat after 15–20 min as necessary
- After patient regains consciousness, provide supplemental carbohydrates asap
- Will not be effective if there is insufficient glycogen stored in the liver
- Stimulates hepatic production of glucose via glycogenolysis
- Can cause tachycardia, nausea, vomiting and hypertension.

10.6 C

The corneal reflex is dependent on the trigeminal and facial nerves.

Method:

- Ask the patient to gaze upwards, and then lightly touch the cornea with a small piece of cotton wool.
- If both eyes blink then the reflex is normal.
- If the patient can feel the touch of the cotton wool it is via the ophthalmic division of the trigeminal nerve, but if there is no reflex blink this is via facial nerve innervation of the orbicularis oculi muscles, which indicates facial nerve palsy. If the patient is unable to feel the touch of the cotton wool, this indicates trigeminal nerve injury.

10.7 E

The prothrombin time is a measure of the integrity of the extrinsic and final common pathways of the coagulation cascade. This consists of tissue factor and factors VII, II (prothrombin), V and X, and fibrinogen. The test is performed by adding calcium and thromboplastin, an activator of the extrinsic pathway, to the blood sample, then measuring the time (in seconds) required for fibrin clot formation.

The reference range for the prothrombin time is 9.5–13.5 s.

The reference range for the international normalised ratio (INR) is <1.3.

10.8 A Yorkshire man who races pigeons presents with a pneumonia. The most likely causative organism is:

A   Chlamydia psittaci

B   Streptococcus pneumoniae

C   Legionella pneumophila

D   Mycoplasma pneumoniae

E   Haemophilus influenzae

10.9 A patient complains of severe chest pain while in the dental chair. Which one of the following is regarded as appropriate management?

A   Administer glucose tablets orally

B   Lie the patient flat

C   Lie the patient in the recovery position

D   Administer intravenous glyceryl trinitrate (GTN)

E   Give the patient oxygen

10.10 Which one of the following statements regarding Down's syndrome is incorrect?

A   It is caused by trisomy 21

B   The incidence increases with the age of the mother

C   Down's patients suffer from microglossia

D   Down's patients suffer from cardiac anomalies

E   Down's patients have delayed eruption of their dentition

10.8 B

In humans, after an incubation period of 5–14 days, the symptoms of the disease range from unapparent illness to systemic illness with severe pneumonia. It presents chiefly as an atypical pneumonia. In the first week of psittacosis the symptoms mimic typhoid fever: prostrating high fevers, arthralgias, diarrhoea, conjunctivitis, epistaxis and leukopenia. Rose spots can appear, called Horder's spots. Splenomegaly develops frequently towards the end of the first week. The diagnosis can be suspected in the case of respiratory infection associated with splenomegaly and/or epistaxis. Headache can be so severe that it suggests meningitis and some nuchal rigidity is not unusual. Towards the end of the first week stupor or even coma can result in severe cases. The infection is treated with antibiotics. Tetracyclines and chloramphenicol are the drugs of choice for treating patients with psittacosis.

10.9 E

Sublingual GTN would be the correct route of administration in a dental setting, not intravenous administration. Glucose would be useful if the patient was hypoglycaemic. Lying the patient flat or in the recovery position may make breathing more difficult for the patient, so this should be avoided.

10.10 C

Down's patients generally have macroglossia. They frequently have congenital cardiac anomalies which require antibiotic cover.

10.11 A 35-year-old smoker has a productive cough with weight loss and drenching night sweats. A chest X-ray shows a right hilar mass with partial collapse of the upper lobe. What is the likely diagnosis?

    A   Pulmonary embolus

    B   Pneumonia

    C   Tuberculosis

    D   Smoker's cough

    E   Asthma

10.12 A 45-year-old alcoholic man is admitted with confusion, ataxia and ophthalmoplegia. He is thin and wasted. What vitamin deficiency does he have?

    A   Vitamin A

    B   Vitamin B_1 (thiamine)

    C   Vitamin B_{12}

    D   Vitamin D

    E   Vitamin K

10.13 Which one of the following is not a feature of congestive cardiac failure?

    A   Breathlessness

    B   Bradycardia

    C   Raised jugular venous pressure

    D   Ankle oedema

    E   Central cyanosis

10.11 C

This is the classic description of tuberculosis. Nodal enlargement is usually unilateral and may cause bronchial compression. Bronchial carcinoma is unlikely in someone so young, but should be ruled out anyway. Pneumonia would be more acute and the patient would have dyspnoea.

10.12 B

This patient has Wernicke's encephalopathy (acute confusion, nystagmus, ataxia, variable ophthalmoplegia), caused by thiamine deficiency. If untreated this will lead to irreversible neurological damage.

10.13 B

As the cardiac output is decreased due to the cardiac failure, the heart rate will increase (tachycardia) to try to make up for this.

10.14 **Which one of the following statements regarding bacterial endocarditis is correct?**

A It does not affect prosthetic heart valves

B It does not occur while using a CPITN probe

C In the UK, it is usually caused by *Streptococcus viridans*

D It may cause a hypochromic microcytic anaemia

E It usually responds well to a 2-week course of amoxicillin

10.15 **Which one of the following statements regarding atrial fibrillation is correct?**

A It is uncommon in elderly people

B It is treated with digoxin

C It does not cause fainting in elderly people

D There is a 'p' wave on an electrocardiogram (ECG)

E The thromboembolic risk is reduced by aspirin more than warfarin

10.16 **Which one of the following statements regarding severe acute asthma is incorrect?**

A The chest is never wheezy

B Both pulse and respiratory rate are high

C Sedation may be used to reduce anxiety

D Nebulised salbutamol may cause muscular tremors

E High percentage oxygen is required

10.14 C

Bacterial endocarditis affects prosthetic heart valves as well as human heart valves. It can occur during any probing procedure, scaling, use of a matrix band or extraction. It can cause a normochromic normocytic anaemia, and requires weeks of intravenous antibiotics to cure it.

10.15 B

Atrial fibrillation is common in elderly people, and is diagnosed on an ECG due to the lack of a 'p' wave. The fibrillation causes fainting in elderly people, and can be treated with digoxin. Warfarin is more efficacious than aspirin at reducing the thromboembolic risk.

10.16 C

Sedation will reduce the respiratory rate, which is entirely the opposite of what is required in severe acute asthma. Oxygen, nebulised salbutamol, steroids and theophyllines are used to treat severe acute asthma.

10.17 Sudden-onset shortness of breath is not associated with which one of the following conditions?

    A Asthma

    B Emphysema

    C Pulmonary embolism

    D Pneumothorax

    E Foreign body inhalation

10.18 Which one of the following is not a feature of chronic liver disease?

    A Spider naevi

    B Ascites

    C Dupuytren's contracture

    D Palmar erythema

    E Pale stools

10.19 Which one of the following statements regarding jaundice is correct?

    A It is always accompanied by dark stools and dark urine

    B It is only caused by viral infections

    C It is associated with pain and weight gain in carcinoma of the pancreas

    D It causes the alanine aminotransferase (ALT) and alkaline phosphatase levels to be reduced

    E It can be associated with post-extraction haemorrhage

10.17 B

Emphysema is a chronic disease that leads to a decrease in lung function over a period of time, but it does not present with an acute shortness of breath.

10.18 E

In chronic liver disease, the patient is likely to have dark stools. They are also likely to have jaundice, weight loss and generalised pruritus.

10.19 E

Not all patients with jaundice have dark stools and dark urine. Jaundice can be also caused by bacterial infection, alcohol, prescription drugs and many other things. Carcinoma of the pancreas is generally painless and is associated with weight loss. ALT and alkaline phosphatase levels tend to increase rather than decrease in jaundice.

10.20 Dysphagia is associated with which one of the following conditions?

    A   Lobar pneumonia

    B   Oesophageal carcinoma

    C   Hyperthyroidism

    D   Hypothyroidism

    E   Atrial fibrillation

10.21 A patient with uncontrolled thyrotoxicosis is unlikely to have:

    A   Increased sweating

    B   Heart block

    C   Resting tremor

    D   Lid retraction

    E   Diarrhoea

10.22 Weight gain is a feature of:

    A   Over-treatment with steroids

    B   Carcinoma of the stomach

    C   Inflammatory bowel disease

    D   Thyrotoxicosis

    E   Chemotherapy

10.20 B

Only in rare circumstances would a thyroid goitre lead to difficulties in swallowing. Oesophageal carcinoma causes progressive dysphagia, and this can have a very rapid onset.

10.21 B

Thyrotoxicosis is likely to cause atrial fibrillation and increased chronotropic rate rather than heart block.

10.22 A

When patients are over-treated with steroids, they have a tendency to have centripetal weight gain. The distribution is known as a buffalo hump, and the patient is described as having a moon face. They are also at risk of osteoporosis, diabetes and immunosuppression.

10.23 Patients who are on dialysis treatment are at risk of:

A   Infections

B   Malnutrition

C   Bleeding diathesis

D   All of the above

E   None of the above

10.24 Which one of the following conditions are renal transplant patients not at risk of?

A   Opportunistic infections

B   Cancer

C   Lymphomas

D   Peptic ulcers

E   Osteoporosis

10.25 One of the physical signs of a left lower motor neurone lesion of the seventh cranial nerve is:

A   Sparing of the muscles of the forehead on the same side

B   An inability to close the right eye

C   Loss of power in the left muscles of mastication

D   Hyperacusis if the nerve to stapedius is involved

E   Decreased sensation over the left maxilla and mandible

10.23 D

Patients who are undertaking dialysis are at risk of infections, malnutrition and bleeding diatheses.

10.24 D

Transplant patients are prescribed steroids and immunosuppressants, which can lead to opportunistic infections and osteoporosis. They are also at an increased risk of cancer, especially lymphomas.

10.25 D

The muscles of mastication and the sensory innervations of the muscles of facial expression are served by the trigeminal nerve. The right eye will not be affected. If it is an upper motor neurone lesion, the muscles of the forehead will be spared. There is hyperacusis when the nerve to stapedius is involved.

10.26 Which one of the following statements regarding trigeminal neuralgia is correct?

A   The pain is continuous

B   The pain involves more than one branch of the trigeminal nerve

C   There is a precise trigger point

D   Dental extraction may help

E   The drug of choice is a steroid

10.27 Which one of the following statements regarding warfarin is true?

A   Warfarin treatment for a pulmonary embolus can be interrupted safely for 1 week when dental treatment is required

B   Warfarin causes reduction of clotting factors II, VII, IX and X

C   Its effects can be reversed by protamine sulphate

D   Bleeding time is the monitoring test for warfarin

E   It has a short life

10.28 Which one of the following is not a cause of a neck lump?

A   Goitre

B   Lymphadenopathy

C   Cystic hygroma

D   Thyroglossal duct cyst

E   Subungual naevus

10.26 C

Trigeminal neuralgia is characterised by an electric shock-like, shooting pain which involves one branch of the trigeminal nerve. There is a trigger point or movement which precipitates the pain. It may be cold wind on the face, or shaving or something like that. Patients often describe this pain as the worst pain imaginable, and find no relief from conventional analgesia. It is treated with carbamazepine, which requires monitoring as it may cause deranged liver function tests and rarely an aplastic anaemia.

10.27 B

Warfarin causes the production of altered clotting factors II, VII, IX and X. It has a long half life of between 48 and 72 hours. It is metabolised in the liver. It is monitored using INR, and patients carry a yellow anticoagulation booklet. It is a teratogenic drug and should be avoided in pregnancy. Protamine sulphate is the reversal agent for heparin. The reversal agent for warfarin is vitamin K.

10.28 E

A subungual naevus is found under the nail of a toe or less commonly a finger, therefore is not found in the neck. It may be a premalignant lesion.

10.29 Which one of the following is not used in the treatment of anaphylaxis?

A   Intramuscular adrenaline injection

B   Intramuscular chlorphenamine injection

C   Hydrocortisone intravenous injection

D   Intravenous diazepam

E   Oxygen

10.30 A patient who weighs 90 kg and is 1 m 82 cm tall has a body mass index of:

A   18

B   21

C   24

D   27

E   30

10.31 Which one of the following circumstances would not raise suspicion of physical abuse in a child?

A   A skull fracture in a 6-week-old baby who allegedly rolled off the bed

B   A torn lingual fraenum in a 2-year-old child

C   Bruises of various ages over the shins of a 6-year-old child

D   Bruises of various ages over the back and buttocks of an 8-year-old child

E   A report by an 8-year-old sibling of an excessive beating

10.29 D

The treatment for anaphylaxis consists of adrenaline, chlorphenamine (anti-histamine), hydrocortisone (steroid), oxygen, intravenous normal saline.

10.30 D

The body mass index is calculated by the weight (in kilograms) divided by the height squared (in metres).

10.31 C

When a child is brought to hospital with an injury, a number of features may raise suspicion of abuse. These include injuries incompatible with the child's age (6-week-old babies cannot roll over), injuries in unusual places and a direct allegation of abuse by the child, a sibling or another adult.

10.32 Which one of the following is a general contraindication to immunisation?

A The presence of coryzal symptoms without significant fever

B A history of a fever up to 38 °C following a previous vaccine

C High-dose corticosteroid therapy when using a live vaccine

D A family history of febrile convulsions

E A history of severe eczema

10.33 Which one of the following statements about chickenpox is incorrect?

A It may be contracted by contact with fluid from vesicles

B It is infectious for 7 days after all vesicles have crusted over

C It is potentially life-threatening in children receiving cancer chemotherapy

D Encephalitis is generally benign and, in most cases, resolves completely

E It is a recognised cause of congenital malformation when the mother is affected in the first 5 months of pregnancy

10.34 Which one of the following statements regarding HIV in children is false?

A In most cases it is due to the administration of contaminated blood products

B It may present with *Pneumocystis pneumoniae*

C It may present with neurological signs in the absence of immunodeficiency

D It is more likely to present with recurrent bacterial infections than in adults

E It may be acquired by breastfeeding from an infected mother

10.32 C

True contraindications to immunisation include acute illnesses, not minor infections without fever or systemic upset. A history of a previous severe local reaction or a severe general reaction within 72 hours of vaccination is a valid contraindication. Live virus vaccines should not be administered to immunosuppressed individuals, including patients receiving high-dose corticosteroids for more than 1 week in the past 3 months, those with malignancies and those receiving chemotherapy.

10.33 B

Varicella virus is spread by respiratory tract droplets or by contact with fluid from vesicles which contain large amounts of virus. Affected individuals cease to be infectious once the last crop of vesicles have dried out. Chickenpox is generally a benign illness but is potentially dangerous to the immunocompromised and to the fetus.

10.34 A

Most HIV infection in children results from vertical transmission from an infected mother. Symptomatic disease presents with infections typical of immunocompromised individuals, but bacterial infection is more common in affected infants than in adults, probably because of the infant's relative immunoglobulin deficiency.

10.35 A 4-month-old boy requires surgery if he is found to have:

   A   A non-retractile foreskin

   B   Bilateral hydrocoeles

   C   A left inguinal hernia

   D   An undescended right testis

   E   An umbilical hernia

10.36 Which one of the following findings make a diagnosis of asthma unlikely?

   A   Lobar collapse identified on a chest X-ray

   B   Cough that only occurs during vigorous exercise

   C   Absence of a family history of asthma

   D   Failure to improve after 2 weeks on high-dose oral steroids

   E   A cough productive of sputum

10.37 In the treatment of asthma:

   A   Most children over 6 years of age can use a metered dose aerosol effectively without a spacer

   B   The use of regular inhaled steroid is limited by a high incidence of side effects

   C   Advice should be given to restrict the child's participation in sport

   D   Oral corticosteroids should be reserved only for children who require hospital admission

   E   Regular anti-inflammatory treatment should be recommended for a child who requires a bronchodilator most days

10.35 C

A non-retractile foreskin is a common finding in pre-school boys. Hydrocoeles and umbilical hernias of varying sizes are a common finding in routine baby checks in the first few months of life. These rarely persist and do not require treatment unless they persist beyond the first year. Inguinal hernias should always be referred for surgery because of the risk of incarceration. If testes are undescended beyond the first year, surgery should be performed.

10.36 D

A central component of asthma is airway inflammation, and if there is no improvement with corticosteroids, the diagnosis should be reconsidered. The inflammation causes hypersecretion of mucus which may lead to lobar collapse by mucus plugging or a productive cough. Although a family history of asthma in children is common, it is not necessary for the diagnosis. Some children's symptoms are exclusively induced by exercise.

10.37 E

Frequent bronchodilator use suggests chronic asthma for which anti-inflammatory treatment would be appropriate. Children (and many adults) have difficulty with the co-ordination required to use metered dose inhalers effectively. Asthmatic children are best treated with inhaled drug delivered via a spacer device or dry metered powder inhaler. The aim of therapy should be to control symptoms to permit a normal life, including participation in sport. Oral corticosteroids are useful in controlling chronic symptoms refractory to inhaled therapy, or in preventing deterioration which would be likely to lead to hospital admission.

10.38 **Which two drugs should be given to a patient you suspect as having myocardial infarction?**

    A   Aspirin and warfarin

    B   Aspirin and paracetamol

    C   Aspirin and clopidogrel

    D   Paracetamol and warfarin

    E   Paracetamol and clopidogrel

10.39 **A 58-year-old woman who has a history of breast cancer presents with jaundice. What is the likely diagnosis?**

    A   Hepatitis B

    B   Metastatic disease

    C   Biliary cirrhosis

    D   Anaemia

    E   Hepatocellular carcinoma

10.40 **A 25-year-old Asian man presents with fever, night sweats and cervical lymphadenopathy. What is the likely diagnosis?**

    A   Oral cancer

    B   Human immunodeficiency virus (HIV) infection

    C   Tuberculosis

    D   Lung cancer

    E   Pneumonia

10.38 C

The correct treatment for a patient suspected of having a myocardial infarction is 300 mg aspirin and 600 mg clopidogrel (Mehta SR. Aspirin and Clopidogrel in Patients with ACS undergoing PCI: CURE and PCI-CURE. *Journal of Invasive Cardiology* 2003;15 Suppl B:17B–20B; discussion 20B–21B).

10.39 B

Breast cancer metastasises to bone and to the liver. Therefore this is the most likely diagnosis. A patient would be unlikely to have had breast cancer and then have a hepatocellular carcinoma.

10.40 C

The most likely diagnosis is tuberculosis. A 25-year-old is unlikely to have a malignancy. The fever, night sweats and lymphadenopathy in a patient of Asian origin is a classical history of tuberculosis.

10.41 A 65-year-old man presents with a markedly raised white cell count and an enlarged spleen. What is the likely diagnosis?

A   Leukaemia

B   Hepatocellular carcinoma

C   Pneumonia

D   Ovarian carcinoma

E   Adenocarcinoma

10.42 A patient has stayed in a hotel for a week and contracts pneumonia. The likely causative organism is:

A   Chlamydia psittaci

B   Streptococcus pneumoniae

C   Legionella pneumophila

D   Mycoplasma pneumoniae

E   Haemophilus influenzae

10.41 A

A patient with splenic enlargement and a markedly raised white cell count is likely to have chronic myeloid leukaemia. The patient is also likely to be tired and have reduced exercise tolerance.

10.42 C

Legionnaire disease is a potentially fatal form of pneumonia that can affect anybody, but which principally affects those who are susceptible because of age, illness, immunosuppression, smoking, etc. It is caused by the bacterium *Legionella pneumophila* and related bacteria that can be found naturally in environmental water sources such as rivers, lakes and reservoirs, usually in low numbers. As they are commonly found in environmental sources they may also be found in purpose-built water systems such as cooling towers, evaporative condensers and whirlpool spas. If conditions are favourable the bacterium may grow creating conditions in which the risk of legionnaire disease is increased.

Index

All references are to chapter and question number